**Places and People Series**

# KEPIER HOSPITAL

by

Dorothy M. Meade

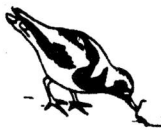

Durham
Turnstone Ventures
1995

© D. M. Meade

1995

ISBN 0 946105 10 3

The publisher wishes to acknowledge with gratitude the financial support of Durham County Council in the production of this book.

# CONTENTS

List of illustrations .................................................................................................iv
Introduction ..........................................................................................................vi
Acknowledgements ..............................................................................................vii
Kepier Hospital
1. The Hospital of St Giles, Durham. ...................................................................1
2. Saint Godric .....................................................................................................3
3. The Hospital in War .........................................................................................3
4. A pilgrim ..........................................................................................................4
5. The Hospital of St Giles of Kepier:
    a new site ........................................................................................................5
    Puiset's endowments ......................................................................................6
    seals ................................................................................................................7
    the borough of St Giles ..................................................................................9
    the parish of St Giles ...................................................................................10
6. The Hospital in its setting ..............................................................................10
7. The Hospital of St Mary .................................................................................13
8. William Wickwane, Archbishop of York, at Kepier ......................................14
9. The Bishops and Kepier:
    Anthony Bek .................................................................................................15
    Letters dated at Kepier .................................................................................15
    Ordinations ...................................................................................................16
10. A corrodian ...................................................................................................16
11. The Scottish War:
    King Edward I ..............................................................................................16
    Queen Isabella ..............................................................................................17
    A fire at Kepier ............................................................................................17
    The depressed state of the Hospital, 1312 ...................................................17
    Disagreement about certain tithes, 1314 .....................................................18
    Depredation by the Scots, 1315 ...................................................................18
12. The buildings at Kepier ................................................................................21
13. The Black Death ...........................................................................................26
14. Poor scholars ................................................................................................26
15. St Nicholas' church and Old Durham ..........................................................27
16. Board and lodging at Kepier ........................................................................27
17. The Masters of Kepier ..................................................................................28
18. The Hospital in 1535 ....................................................................................31
19. The closing of the Hospital ..........................................................................33
20. Lay owners: ..................................................................................................36
    John Cockburn .............................................................................................37
    The Heath Family .........................................................................................38
    The Cole Family ..........................................................................................44
    The Musgrave Family ..................................................................................45
        Kepier Gardens ......................................................................................45
        Two artists at Kepier ..............................................................................46
        Kepier Inn ..............................................................................................47
        Kepier mill .............................................................................................49
        The last of the gardens and the inn ........................................................52
        Lepers? ...................................................................................................52
        The North Eastern Electricity Board .....................................................54
21. An end in tranquillity ...................................................................................54
Appendix: notes on illustrations .........................................................................57
List of abbreviations ...........................................................................................62
Documents in Durham County Record Office ...................................................63
Notes and references ...........................................................................................64

# Illustrations

Front cover: Kepier Gatehouse, west front, today.

Inside front cover: Descent of Heath of Kepier.

Frontispiece: *Fading Grandeur*, etching *c.* 1900. ...............viii
1. Kepier Farm: plan of location. ................v
2. St Giles' church, late 18th century. ................1
3. Kepier Hospital seal, 1335. ................8
4. Tithe Barn, photograph before demolition. ................11
5. Tithe Barn, High Grange, before 1964: plan and elevation. ........11
6. St Mary Magdalen Hospital, 1846. ................13
7. Kepier Farm site: plan. ................20
8. Kepier Hospital, 1595. ................21
9. Kepier Gateway, west face, 1846. ................21
10. Kepier Gateway, shields on west front. ................22
11. Kepier Gateway, carved corbels. ................22
12. Kepier farmhouse, facing east. ................23
13. Kepier Gateway: east face. ................24
14. Kepier farmhouse: sculptured crucifixion. ................24
15. Carved head (corbel?) 15th century layman. ................25
16. Heath coat of arms. ................39
17. Houghton-le-Spring old grammar school:
    Heath and Gilpin inscription, 1724. ................40
18. Houghton-le-Spring old grammar school:
    Tempest commemorative inscription, 1777. ................40
19. St Giles' church: recumbent effigy of John Heath, *d.*1590. ........41
20. Kepier: panorama view (S.H. Grimm, 1777-84) ................42
21. Heath mansion, S. and W. elevations, 1883-8. ................43
22. Kepier garden plan, O.S. 1858. ................46
23. Heath mansion from the north-west, *c.*1887. ................47
24. Bricked-up gateway to Heath mansion grounds. ................48
25. Blocked window in west wall of Kepier mansion. ................48
26a. Kepier: general view, late 19th century. ................50
26b. River Wear at Kepier looking downstream, 1994 ................51
27. Kepier mill: arch over mill-race. ................51
28a. Remains of the mansion house today. ................53
28b. Kepier mansion house ruin: plan. ................53
29. Gatehouse, east side, *c.*1930. ................55
30a. Kepier Farm: east side, south end. ................56
30b. Kepier Farm: east side, north end ................56

Inside back cover: Descent of Cole of Gateshead, Kepier and Brancepeth.

Back cover: Watercolour of west side of Gatehouse, 1774-8.

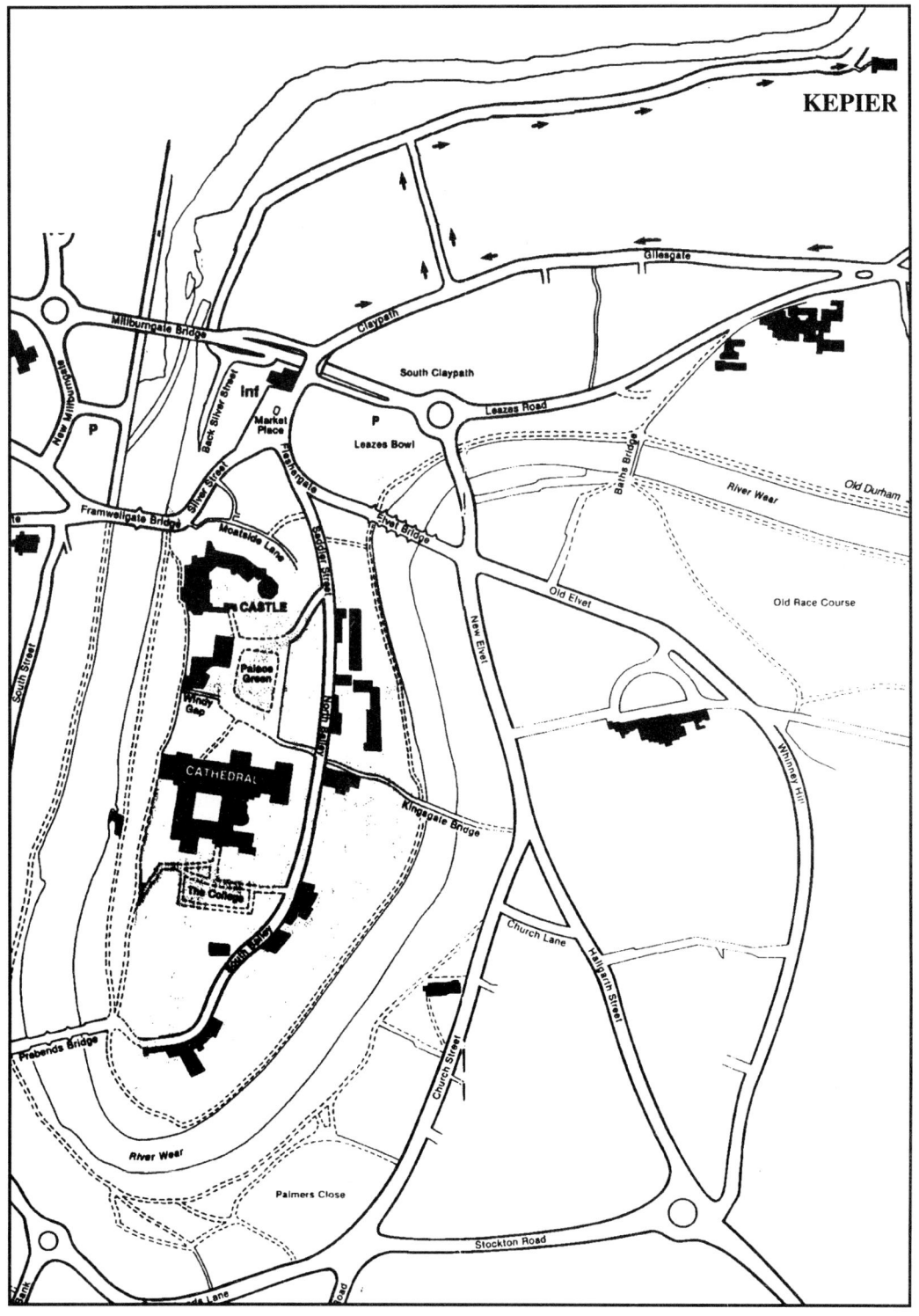

*Robin Taylor Wilson*

Kepier: plan showing location.

# Introduction

Kepier Hospital, or more properly the Hospital of St Giles of Kepier, once held an important place in the life of Durham. At the time it was founded, St Giles Church was the Hospital chapel and lay close to a great highway which brought travellers from the South, crossed the high ridge beyond the top of Gilesgate bank, descended to cross the River Wear and mounted the opposite hill in the direction of Newton (Hall) and led north to Newcastle. The roads to Sherburn and Sunderland were developed primarily to connect Durham Priory with its estates at Pittington and, more distantly, at Wearmouth, after the Community of St Cuthbert settled on the Durham Peninsula in 995.

Forty years after the first Hospital buildings were destroyed in 1144, a new site was chosen near the same great highway, but close to the river crossing. This was an excellent position both for the many travellers on the road, and for pilgrims who turned aside here to visit the shrine of St Cuthbert at Durham. An institution of this type always welcomed strangers. The accommodation was good and could provide even for occasioal royal visitors. The way into Durham from Kepier lay along the bank of the Wear, past the freemen's pasture called The Sands, and so to the foot of Walkergate also known as Back Lane, or, more significantly, the "way to Kepier". Walkergate, a steep street which descended from the (now vanished) Clayport Gate, alongside the city wall on the north side of St Nicholas church, was demolished in 1964 to make way for the approach to Milburngate Bridge. To reach Kepier today on foot by the riverside route, there is a choice between the footpaths reached from Back Silver Street, and from the foot of Providence Row. The latter is also suitable for cars. Beyond the Sands on the left, and a residential development on the right, lie the remains of Kepier, its gatehouse facing the river. Here, the road peters out into a field path. It is difficult to imagine that just beyond Kepier a busy main road once carried a stream of traffic. The great highway has vanished, and Kepier gatehouse stands dreaming by the waterside. The fascinating story of Kepier comes alive in the following pages. The people who knew it as a hospital, a gentleman's residence, an inn with pleasure gardens, or latterly as a farm and private house, are traced in a delightful narrative derived from extensive and careful research, which is well illustrated by maps, prints, photographs and drawings. Dorothy Meade has greatly enriched our knowledge not only of Kepier, but of Durham itself.

Margot Johnson *(editor)*.

# Acknowledgements

I am grateful for the help of the staffs of Durham Dean and Chapter Library (Mr Roger Norris); Durham University Library (especially Mrs Linda Drury); Durham City Library; and the Durham Record Office. Assistance of varying kinds was also given by Mr Michael F. Richardson, Mr Martin Roberts, Mr Martin Taylor, Mr Robin Taylor-Wilson and others mentioned in the notes. In addition I should like to record my gratitude to the editor for her guidance and helpful suggestions.

Finally I wish to thank Mrs Ruth Watson for welcoming me on frequent visits to Kepier and sharing my own enthusiasm for the history of the hospital.

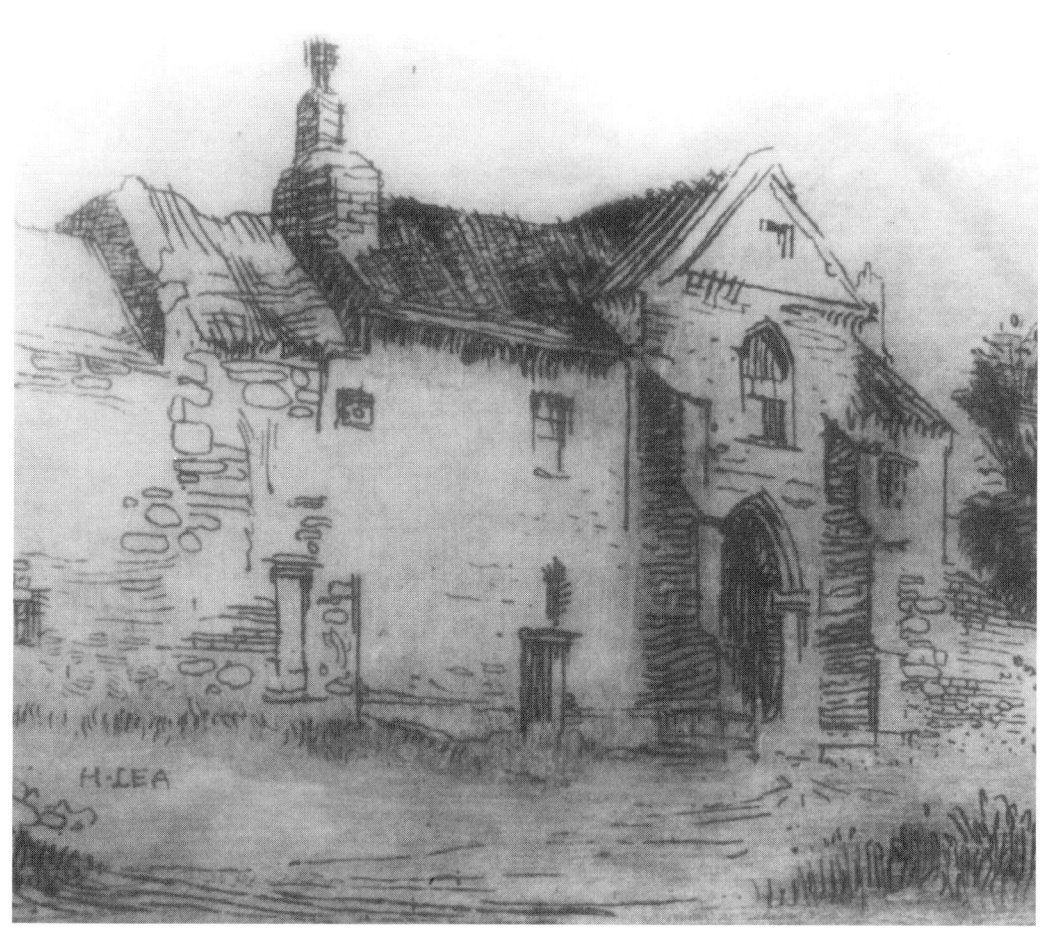

*H. Lea*

Frontispiece: *Fading Grandeur*, etching *c.* 1900

# Kepier Hospital

## 1. THE HOSPITAL OF ST GILES, DURHAM

The first site of the Hospital of St Giles, Durham, was at the top of the hill now called Gilesgate. This was about three-quarters of a mile north-east of the cathedral, beside the only road that led into the city without having to cross the river Wear. It was near the junction of three well-used roads - that from the manors of the Prior and Convent at Wearmouth, one from Pittington and another from Sherburn and the south-east. A water-supply was available as it would be easy to sink a well in this glacial sand and gravel site. A Holy Well, perhaps so-called because of its connection with the hospital, remained in use till the end of the nineteenth century. It was some 200 yards east of the hospital church.

There were then about thirty-two hospitals in England and this was the first one to be built in County Durham. It was founded by Bishop Rannulf Flambard (1099-1128) as an almshouse for the 'keeping of the poor who enter the same hospital'. These would be feeble old men who were unable to work any more.

Flambard dedicated the hospital church on 11 June 1112. In his charter he said 'I have made this church in honour of God and St Giles'. This was one of the earliest examples of a popular hospital dedication. It was especially apt, as the French saint was thought of as

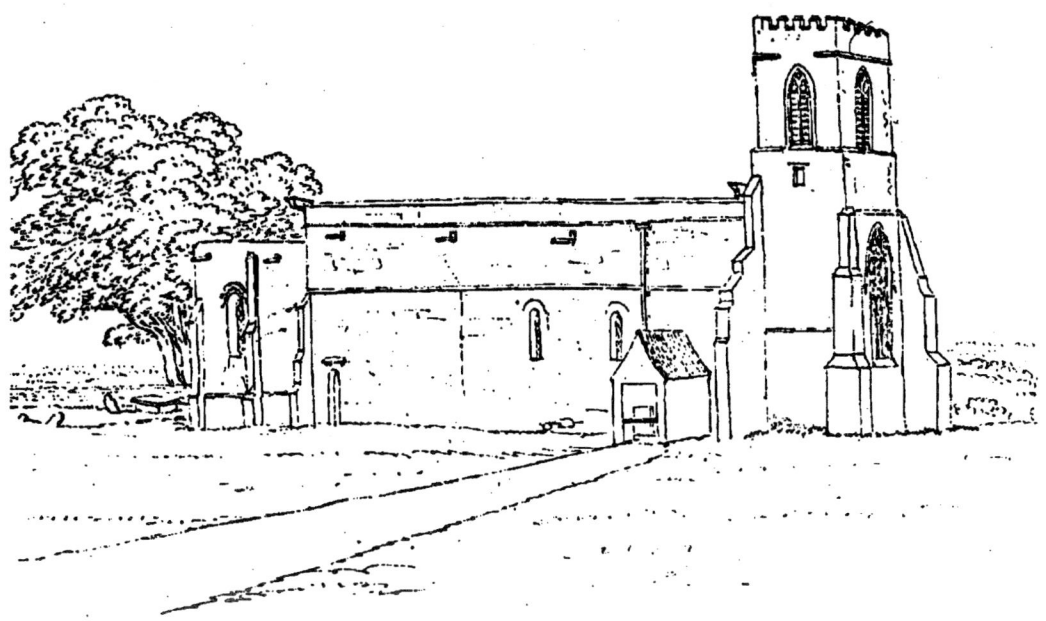

*S. H. Grimm (1777-84)*

2. St. Giles' Church, Durham.

the patron of beggars and cripples, although he was probably an imaginary figure, invented in the south of France to take advantage of the pilgrims travelling to Compostella.[1] He was supposed to have been shot in the leg by an arrow when a hind fled to him while trying to escape from a royal hunt; consequently he limped ever after. Some of the later hospital seals show the saint, carrying a crozier and book, with his hind looking up at him.

Flambard, acknowledging that he was a 'sinner and unworthy', gave the hospital for the health of his own soul and for the redemption of the souls of the Norman kings of England. He also remembered 'the souls of those who have given anything in alms to the Church of St Cuthbert' (i.e. the cathedral). This was obvious encouragement for pilgrims to visit St Cuthbert's shrine and suggests that Flambard had them and their donations in mind, as well as the aged poor, when he founded his hospital. They would receive supper, bed and breakfast there for whatever payment they could afford.

The living quarters were almost certainly wooden or wattle-and-daub structures.

Some of them probably fronted the road, having a wide gateway giving access to a large yard, with the church on the far side. This would explain the fact that the church is set back from the road and not easily seen by passers-by. Built of stone, it is the only part to survive to the present time (with additions and alterations). Until recently it has always been thought to have consisted of a nave and chancel of the same width. It has now been put forward, as 'a plausible alternative', that the nave may have been originally an infirmary hall with a crossing or tower at its east end, and the actual chapel beyond that.[2] Whatever its plan it would have been the centre of communal life, with more care and money being lavished on it than on any other part of the hospital.

The only member of staff mentioned in the charter was a clerk (i.e. a priest). He would have supervised the running of the house with a number of lay assistants. His main task was thought to be the daily celebration of mass and the reciting of the canonical hours at certain intervals throughout the day, for the routine was primarily religious. The name of only one clerk is known: in 1131 Meldred, 'priest of St Giles' [hospital]' was a witness (with many others) to a charter of the Prior and Convent granting land to Dolfin (ancestor of the Nevilles of Raby).[3]

The inmates were expected to attend the devotions in the church for the sake of their souls. Little could be done for the health of their bodies other than providing them with food and rest, warmth and cleanliness. Some of them were, perhaps, chronic invalids, but others would be able to do odd jobs about the place. They could expect to stay for a few years only, at the most, before death overtook them.[4]

Flambard endowed the hospital with his village of Caldecotes, which, with its plains, pastures, meadows, woods, water and land, both cultivated and uncultivated, was clearly a thriving place. It probably touched the city boundary on the west and the river Wear on its northern and southern edges so that the hospital was built on village land. By 1430 it was referred to as 'the manor of Caldecotes, called Kypiyer Grange'.[5] The main inhabited part seems to have been about three-quarters of a mile north-east of the hospital in the area of the later High Grange. Flambard also granted a mill on the Millburn (at Durham).[6] As an additional food supply, he directed that every year two sheaves [from each thrave of the corn tithe] should be sent to the hospital by fifteen of his own villages. No dues were demanded for these gifts, which were made in 'free and perpetual alms' (i.e. no military service was required as a condition of holding them).[7]

The income from the endowments enabled the hospital to perform its duties of caring for the poor and receiving guests 'as if they were Christ Himself'.[8]


## 2. SAINT GODRIC

At some time between 1112 and 1128 Godric, a former seafaring merchant adventurer, came to the hospital. During his voyages he had visited many of the holy places of Christendom, including the island of Farne. Inspired, perhaps, by the story of Cuthbert, who had lived there, he decided to settle down in Durham where the saint was buried. There he went to the hospital church of St Giles daily and was appointed to the position of doorkeeper, the lowest of the minor orders of the Western Church. His duties would have been similar to those of a modern verger. Eventually he left the city to become a hermit in the secluded woods at Finchale. Soon he acquired a reputation as a worker of miracles and his fame reached even Thomas Becket and the pope. After his death in 1170 local people thought of him as a saint. Many pilgrims resorted to his grave at Finchale, especially women, who were denied entrance to St Cuthbert's shrine at Durham.[9]


## 3. THE HOSPITAL IN WAR [10]

When Bishop Geoffrey Rufus died in 1140 Durham became embroiled in a serious Anglo-Scottish conflict. Because of its advantageous position overlooking the city the hospital was involved in the disturbances that followed.

The border between England and Scotland was not clearly defined at that time and, on the death of the bishop, the Scottish king, David I, saw an opportunity of extending his influence as far as the river Tees. He therefore supported the efforts of his own chancellor, William Cumin, a man well-known in Durham, to become the next bishop.

Cumin had no difficulty in taking control of the diocese, having won over most of the barons of the bishopric. The monks, who possessed the right of election, refused to accept him and after two unhappy years some of them managed to escape to York. There they elected William of St Barbara, dean of York, as their lawful bishop.

In the summer of 1143 the Bishop and his retinue rode north to the castle at Bishopton, near Sedgefield, which belonged to Roger Conyers, the only baron of the bishopric who had not paid homage to Cumin. From there he and the faithful Conyers, with other barons who had decided to join them, advanced towards Durham, via the Sherburn road, accompanied by a considerable body of troops. They went first to the Hospital of St Giles, which they intended to use as a base, and surrounded the church with a rampart, 'so as to have that place for their defence.' Only after that was an approach made to the castle, but the men were driven back 'as if they had been enemies.' Retreating to the church of St Giles, 'at some little distance from the walls,' the Bishop and his company spent the night there.

Further attempts to enter the city in peace failed so, rather than risk more bloodshed, William of St Barbara ordered a return to Bishopton 'although he was in a position to have offered resistance.' The occupants of the hospital were doubtless relieved to see them go, despite the fact that they themselves remained dangerously close to the determined chancellor and his savage adherents.

At the beginning of 1144 the bishop, fearing for his life, withdrew to Lindisfarne. By this time it had become increasingly obvious to King David that his candidate, although in possession at Durham, would never be recognised as bishop. He therefore offered assistance to William of St Barbara and in August the bishop rode south with a large military escort under the command of the Scottish king's heir. This host drew near to Durham, probably by fording the river Wear at some point north or north-east of the hospital of St Giles. Even then, William Cumin was unwilling to submit. He sent out a contingent of his henchmen to set fire to the Hospital, so preventing the bishop seeking refuge there as he had done in the previous year. The inhabitants must have fled in terror to the stone church which was the only place of safety.

Cumin's men also 'burnt to the ground the entire vill which belonged to [the hospital]', i.e. Caldecotes. The advancing army would have found food and fodder there, so it was an obvious target for the opposing force.

The usurper continued his resistance for a time but finally realised that his cause was lost. On 18 October the Bishop entered the city to receive Cumin's submission. The defeated intruder promised 'that he would make satisfaction for every injury that he had inflicted upon any one.' This statement gave hope that the hospital, among other victims, could expect to receive some compensation for the damage done to it. Being an episcopal foundation the Bishop probably made sure that reparations were made so that reconstruction could begin.

## 4. A PILGRIM

In the latter half of the twelfth century many stories of miracle cures at Durham and Finchale were written down by Reginald, a monk of Durham. One incident was about a Norwegian lad who had suffered from a strange disorder in the head for seven years. A bishop recommended his mother and father to cast lots in order to find out which of three English saints, Cuthbert, Edmund or Thomas Becket, possessed the greatest power. The parents having done so, the lot of Cuthbert was declared victorious. Therefore, in April 1172, the afflicted youth was brought to Durham by his brother. They stayed in the 'hospital which is situated outside the walls of the city', and this must have been St Giles'. At dawn the next day they went to the cathedral where the elder gave an account of the troubles of the younger one to the guardian of the shrine. The monks offered intercessions to St Cuthbert on behalf of the sufferer and that night he was allowed to remain at the tomb in vigil, praying for mercy. In the early morning the monks found him 'extremely fit, rubicund, seeing, hearing and holding his head up in a perfectly natural way.'

People at the hospital must have been amazed to see the sick person who had left them the day before returning in good health. It was a privilege for them to have witnessed this demonstration of the might of the holy Cuthbert.

## 5. THE HOSPITAL OF ST GILES OF KEPIER

### A new site

It may have been in the hope of attracting more pilgrims that, about 1180, Bishop Hugh of Le Puiset (1154-95) refounded the hospital on a different site. This was half a mile north of the old one beside the river Wear at Kepier. The name 'Kepier' is made up of two Old English words giving the meaning 'weir with a fish trap'.[11] In time the two words merged to become a place-name, so that the new establishment was henceforth known as the Hospital of St Giles of Kepier or, more simply, Kepier Hospital. As a fishery was not mentioned in Flambard's charter, the weir with its trap (or basket) may have been constructed since 1112. The convenience of being nearer the supply of fish, a common item in the diet of those days (especially during Lent), possibly prompted the move. There is no medieval record of the types of fish caught. One example would have been salmon which was given to the lepers at Sherburn hospital (two miles distant) on St Cuthbert's day in Lent, if it could be procured.

Sandstone was available at Kepier quarry about a mile north-east of the proposed location, where the river flows through a deep gorge. This is the same place which, by local tradition, provided much of the stone for the building of Durham cathedral.[12]

The remodelled institution was built on a generous scale and included an infirmary, a church, a dormitory, a hall and a court below which confessions were to be heard (perhaps a crypt-chapel). A master appointed by the Bishop was head of the establishment. The staff was made up of thirteen brethren called conversi,[13] the most senior of whom appears to have been known as the prior. All were under the usual monastic vows. Six were chaplains (one acting as confessor), bound to pray for the souls of Flambard and Puiset; they would celebrate mass, sing the daily services and render any religious assistance required. The others were lay brethren who were assigned work concerned with the running of the hospital and its lands: the seventh brother was a steward whose duties included looking after the food supplies; the eighth was in charge of the tannery; the ninth was a baker; the tenth, a miller; the eleventh, the granger, supervised the agricultural estates and was keeper of the ploughs; the twelfth managed the livestock; and the thirteenth, the receiver and attorney-general, directed the business and legal affairs of the hospital. Should the staff increase to more than thirteen at some future time the master could then, with the consent of the prior and brethren, assign suitable posts to the newcomers.

The brethren led a life in common: they shared a table in the hall 'unless the master, for the accommodation of guests, or other honest cause, should at any time order otherwise'; they slept in the dormitory unless they were ill, when they were sent to the infirmary. Every year they were given a new habit. It must have been a distinctive dress for, in 1244, Nicholas Farnham, bishop of Durham, decided that the staff of the Hospital of St James, Northallerton (founded 1197-1208) should adopt the habit of the brethren of Kepier. The chaplains were allowed two pairs of boots a year; the labouring brethren, who had more strenuous work to do, could have footgear of a stouter type as often as they needed them. Household articles, such as cloth for bedding, were supplied when the prior thought them necessary.

The number of inmates to be maintained was not stated. In 1244 Farnham provided for thirteen at Northallerton. Since this had a staff similar in size to that of Kepier it seems probable that there were at least thirteen inmates at the Durham hospital. These would be old men as there were no sisters on the staff.[14] St James' also gave lodging to thirteen poor people each night. Kepier, in a busy pilgrimage centre, may have taken in a greater number of travellers and pilgrims for bed and breakfast.[14]

## Puiset's endowments

After confirming Flambard's donations, Puiset issued three charters by means of which he bestowed lands, goods and rights on the hospital.

The village of Clifton, with its lands, waters, mills and fisheries, was part of the endowment. It seems to have been near Low Grange Farm, Belmont, where fields called High Clifton and Low Clifton are marked on the tithe map (1846). In 1331 it was described, with Caldecotes, as being 'on the east part of the hospital of Kypier'. It would therefore be adjacent to Caldecotes.

The greater part of the corn-rent for alms in Durham was now paid to the hospital. Puiset granted a toft (probably as a temporary store for the corn) in each village that owed it tithes, namely, Houghton, Ryhope, Easington, Darlington, Sedgefield, Boldon and Whickham. If Darlington has been written in error for Quarrington, then these are seven of the fifteen villages mentioned by Flambard in 1112 as obliged to give two sheaves every year to the hospital. It would seem that, in the intervening years, the sheaves of these seven had been increased to a tithe, while those of the others, save those of Newton, had been granted elsewhere, presumably in some satisfactory exchange. Flambard's remaining sheaves were parted with in 1189 when an agreement was made with the Prior and Convent that the hospital could retain the tithes of Clifton, formerly payable to the church of St Oswald in Durham. In return, the hospital consented to make a yearly offering of one bezant or two shillings on the altar of St Oswald's on its saint's day and, in addition, to release to that church the two sheaves of Newton. Puiset also gave the tithes of his demesne lands (i.e. lands which he kept in his own hands and did not grant away) recently brought into cultivation, in his own diocese, as well as elsewhere in the province of York including Howden parish (East Riding).[15]

Thraves were an endowment in grain (24 sheaves, usually wheat) distinct from tithe. Puiset granted a thrave of corn from every carucate (ploughland) of his demesne, 'just as is given to the hospital of St Peter in Yorkshire'. The latter received the thraves of every carucate in the diocese of York and these formed more than half of its revenues. Similarly, the thraves paid to Kepier must have been a substantial part of its income. They were known as 'gillycorn' (or 'Saintgilicorn' or 'le gelycorne').

The new hospital church at Kepier was dedicated to St Mary and All Saints. For the purpose of roofing it and the infirmary Puiset, in his third charter, gave a lead-mine in

Weardale. This linking of church and infirmary suggests that they were both under one roof. If so, the bed-ridden old men, cared for in the sick-ward at the west end, would have been able to hear mass and prayers being said in the church. This arrangement, possibly repeating Flambard's plan, became a model for some later hospitals and almshouses.[16] The grant of an iron-mine at Rookhope, also in Weardale, was to supply iron for making ploughs. A peat-bog at Newton, on the opposite side of the river from the hospital, would provide fuel.

At Hunstanworth, north of Rookhope, the hospital held 'a certain assart [land which had until recently been waste] and pasture for the feeding of cattle and beasts for the use of the poor, which the lord bishop gave to them in alms.' This was near the bishop's hunting park in Weardale, where the strict Norman forest laws insisted that the forefeet of dogs kept in the forest should be maimed to prevent them chasing the game. Since wolves roamed the west Durham fells and domestic animals had to be protected from them, Puiset waived the law on condition that the herdsmen of the hospital kept their dogs leashed.

By these gifts of property and produce made by Puiset the hospital was liberally endowed and clearly favoured by the Bishop. This encouraged others to follow his example for, in return, prayers would be said in the hospital church for the souls of themselves and their families - a matter of great importance, according to the religious beliefs of the time. Gilbert, Puiset's chamberlain, for instance, held land at Kepier and gave permission for the master and brethren to make their mill-dam and mill-pool there. Gilbert Hansard, one of the barons of the bishopric, gave his village of Amerston, near Hartlepool, and land in Hurworth, near Darlington; this substantial donation was made in order to support an additional chaplain who would pray forever for the souls of himself, his father and mother and all his kin.

Endowments continued to be made in subsequent years so that the hospital gained many scattered possessions in land, varying from twelve acres at Medomsley to all Walter de Witton's land at Frosterley. They also included the mill at Crawcrook and a fishery on the Tyne.

Besides these means of support Puiset's second charter spared the hospital certain customary payments, whether to the bishop, the archdeacon, the dean or other officials. It was thus in a privileged position and enabled to grow in wealth and influence.

### Seals[17]

Examples of five different types of seals in use at Kepier Hospital have survived. The earliest is attached to a document of 1189. Pointed oval in shape (as are the other seals of the hospital), it is in green wax. The only symbol is a cross with two bars (or cross patriarchal) and round the edge are the words (in Latin), 'Seal of Saint Giles'. Ten years later, on a seal of white wax, the cross is similar to that used on the seal of the cathedral priory, i.e. with slender arms widened at the ends; the inscription has now become, 'Seal of Saint Giles of Durham'. Not until the years 1219-33 does the figure of St Giles appear, on a green seal; he is wearing a monastic habit, holding a book and a crosier, and the hind is looking up at him; the words are now, 'Seal of Saint Giles of Kepier'. Another seal, in white wax, of 1291, is similar. On the back of this one is a small, oval secretum (or privy

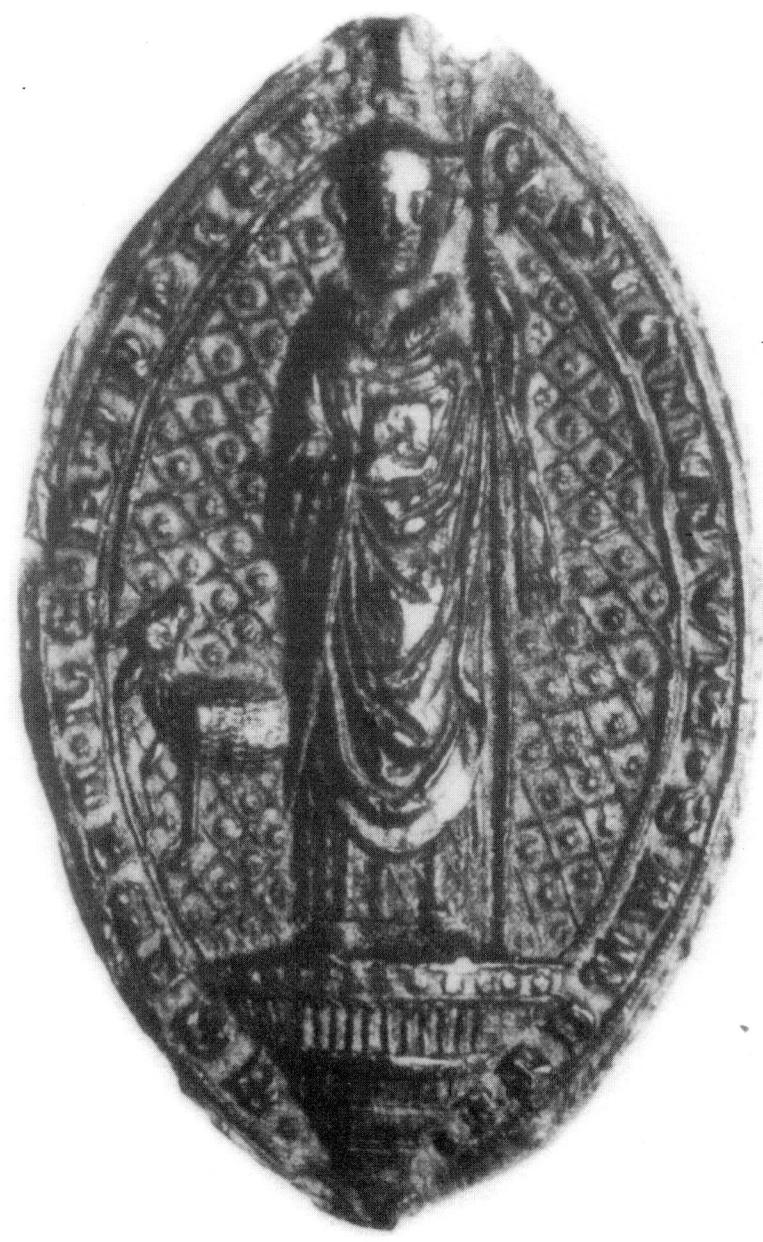

3. Seal of Kepier Hospital, 1335.

seal), a gem with an inscribed shape on it, possibly that of a lion. This was probably used for private letters. The words, 'Frange, Lege, Tege' round the margin may mean 'Break, Select, Protect'. The finest seal, in black wax, is attached to a document of 1335. Here, St Giles is standing on a bracket and wearing mass vestments, against a diamond-patterned background. This was still being used in 1352. These seals would have been appended to the hospital's charters and other important documents to authenticate them.

## The borough of St Giles

In his first charter Puiset said, 'We grant to this same master and brethren and to all their men to whom they concede liberty a free burgage in the vicus of St Giles, Durham'. A vicus was a very small unwalled town or village, often met with on the continent at that time, outside a walled town. It might also be known as a borough, as was St Giles'. There is no evidence, up to this time, of any settlement near the first hospital. It would therefore seem that the master and brethren would create the vicus, and that the borough of St Giles was a planned town. Naturally, it was sited at the top of the hill beside the road leading into Durham, and near the former hospital church which became a parish church to serve the new community. Gradually it developed down the hill to the west so that, in time, it linked up with the city of Durham itself.

The houses of a vicus were built along a street. North Row and South Row are mentioned in the vicus of St Giles in 1539. These are still apparent on either side of the road, but set back from it to allow for an open space, approximately rectangular in shape, about 250 yards long. This would have served quite adequately for a market. Although there was no grant of one in the charter, the master and brethren perhaps hoped to obtain one, as did the Prior and Convent for their borough in Elvet. It seems that the bishop denied this privilege to both boroughs for the protection of his own market at Durham.

It would be an advantage for the hospital to have craftsmen and traders living in burgages (houses with long strips of land behind) near at hand. These skilled men could supply it with goods which the villeins had no opportunity to produce. Some of the burgesses (townsmen) may have been freed villeins from Caldecotes and Clifton. It was a condition of their tenure that the new burgesses should perform certain agricultural services, for they had to abide by the custom of Kepier and so were not entirely free. The most common of these was helping with the harvest on Kepier's demesne land in the autumn (usually for three 'boon-days'). Many of the St Giles' burgages are still in existence as their boundaries would always be jealously guarded.

Although Puiset's charter provided for an incipient borough with burgage tenements, it granted no strong borough privileges to the future burgesses. The master and brethren were given the right to hold a court, i.e. a manorial court with jurisdiction over the burgesses, denying them their own self-governing borough court. Its meeting-place was located in the main street: on Monday 18 January 1373/74 the grant of a burgage, 'in the vicus of St Giles', mentioned 'the house of Kypier called the Curthous' adjacent to it.

The hospital and its burgesses were allowed some useful advantages: no-one could take 'distress' from them (i.e. seize and hold goods legally, probably as a result of debt); there was no requirement to provide men for armed service[18] and they were to be exempt from certain taxes and dues; firewood, timber and fencing could be taken from the bishop's land, where it could be obtained easily but without waste; and they were able to pasture their swine in any of the bishop's forests. All of these benefits were meant to induce people to come and settle in the borough in order to form a little trading community.

To the new townsmen the borough, with its own court, church and customs, was their home; and the usual customary rents were paid to its overlord, the Master of Kepier. They thought of themselves as men of the borough of St Giles rather than as citizens of Durham;

in 1242, when the king's justices visited Durham, the 'men of the vicus of St Giles' paid them sixty shillings, as a body, 'so that they would not be troubled'. This was preferred to having their affairs probed into with consequent loss of time and possible fines. Only with the passing of the medieval centuries did their successors feel that they lived in 'the suburbs of the city of Durham'.[19]

### The parish of St Giles

The parish of St Giles was formed at this time. It comprised the hospital's villages of Clifton and Caldecotes and stretched from the boundary with St Nicholas' parish on the west to that of Pittington parish on the east, a distance of some two and three-quarter miles. This was a large tract of land identical with that of the manor of St Giles. Flambard's original church became the parish church and its font probably dates from this time. To accommodate the incoming population Puiset extended it by adding a new chancel. The church was appropriated to the hospital, i.e. the hospital became the rector, receiving at least two-thirds of the income of the parish from oblations and tithes. The hospital also had the advowson (the right to appoint a vicar) and would have put in a chaplain at a small stipend. Richard of the Vicus of St Giles was named as the parochial chaplain in 1314.

The church became the centre of life in the borough and all the residents attended it every Sunday and on religious festivals, as well as for the family occasions of baptisms, marriages and funerals that punctuated their lives.

As the main street led from the city to or past the church it became known as Saintgilligate (gata - or gate - being an Old Norse word meaning 'a road'), or just Gilligate (later, Gilesgate).

## 6. THE HOSPITAL IN ITS SETTING

The hospital lay towards the western end of its Durham property and about half a mile north of the main community dwellings, with the river running past its west-facing entrance. In spite of the secluded site 'the poor and strangers constantly resorting thither' were attracted to it. From the city it could be approached by either of two roads, each branching off Claypath (the road which eventually joined Gilesgate) to the north. One was named in deeds early in the fourteenth century to locate the positions of burgages. In 1340 William de Whalton was given the lease of a tenement in Durham near 'the highway which leads to the Hospital of Kippeyar and to the Chapel of St Thomas the Martyr'. The road indicated would seem to be the one now called Providence Row. The other ('the Bakehouse Lane, otherwise Back Lane, otherwise Walker's Gate') led from Claypath immediately east of the market place. In October 1617 it was referred to as the road 'from Durham to Kepier and beyond'. At that time 'the stretch between the [bishop's] bakehouse and the bishop's mills was in dangerous decay' and the parishioners of St. Nicholas' were ordered to repair it.[20] Visitors and pilgrims staying in the hospital, as well as members of the staff, must have used these routes frequently.

The manor was managed for its agricultural resources. Kepier Lane connected the hospital with Caldecotes and Clifton. Apparently the two villages were partially depopulated in order to be worked as granges, some of the villeins being kept as farm labourers. In a charter of 1331 they are referred to as 'their manors of Caldecots and Clyftone . . . which now are called granges'. By the end of the sixteenth century they had acquired the distinguishing titles of West and East or Hither and Far (later High and Low) Granges respectively, and these topographical names may have grown into use in earlier centuries.

After the gathering of the harvest the corn was carted to Kepier from the many villages that owed tithes and thraves to the hospital. As they brought their produce at the same time of the year there was always difficulty in storing it. This problem was overcome in the thirteenth or fourteenth century by the building of a tithe barn at Caldecotes. It was a large, sturdy, stone structure, measuring approximately 47m. long, 10m. wide and 9m. high. In

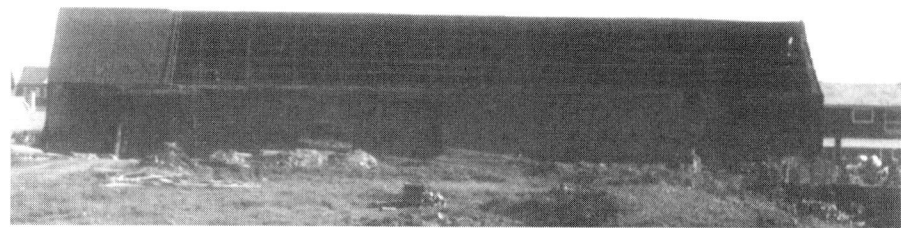

*Photograph by L. S. K. Le Fleming*

4. Tithe Barn before demolition.

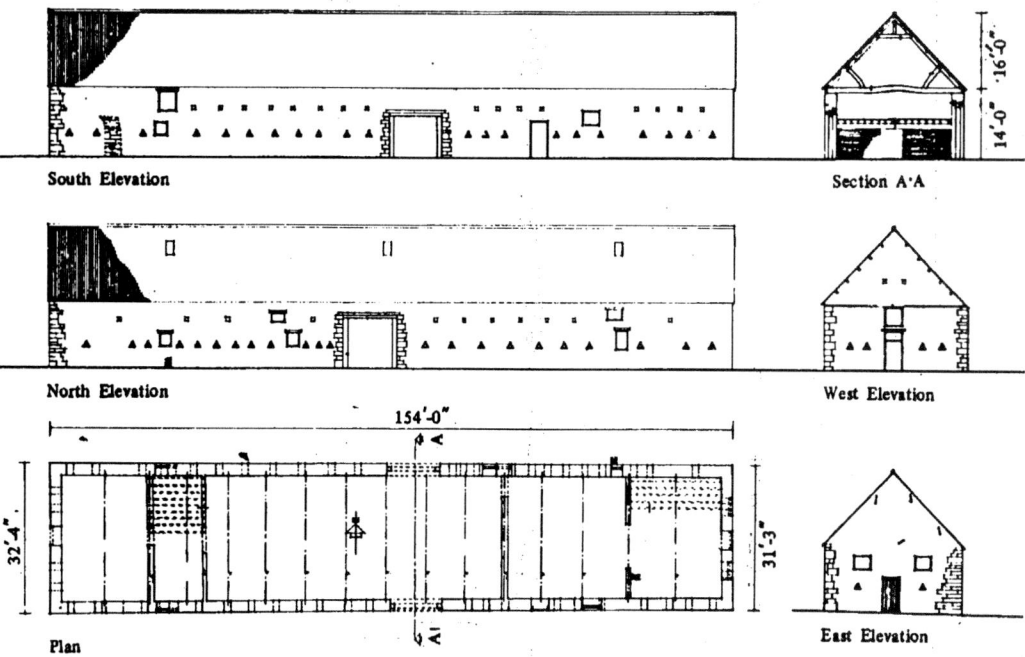

*Drawing by D. Staines*

5. Tithe Barn, High Grange, before 1964, plan and elevation.

the centre of each long wall was a gateway, about 3m high and wide, to allow the horses and carts to enter before unloading began.[21] The annual coming and going of the big wagons provided a contact with a wider world for both the drivers and the St Giles' parishioners. Possibly the visitors - those who could afford it - took home with them a useful object made and bought in the borough - a leather purse, perhaps, a length of woollen cloth or a wooden bowl.

The paths to the hospital from Gilesgate and clusters of houses throughout the parish were well-trodden. The reapers, who had gathered in their own corn, carried it, when needed, on backs or in wheelbarrows, down to Kepier to be ground in the hospital's mill. For this service they had to pay a proportion of the meal to the master and brethren as a manorial obligation. The hospital had a further claim on its tenants: when the bread mixture was ready the housewives were required to take it to the common ovens, where the loaves were baked on payment of a small charge. A tenement behind the bakehouse of St Giles' street belonged to Agnes Hextildesham in 1330. The bakehouse was the first house on the north side of Gilesgate and it has given its name to the adjacent lane.[22]

At regular intervals the master of the hospital, or his deputy, came to the court-house in the borough, perhaps reaching it by the vennel opposite the church, in order to preside over the manor court. A chaplain probably accompanied him to note the proceedings although only one pre-Reformation court book survives, covering the period 1494-1532. Some of the court's time was given to the surrendering of tenements and the admittance of new tenants, whose titles were entered on the court roll. Also, details of petty misdemeanours and offences against manor regulations were heard and punishments, usually small fines, imposed; for instance, in 1528 a tenant was fined for cutting and carrying away trees or wood for firewood from Kepier's demesne land. The business over, the master returned down the slope to the hospital, with his chaplain bearing the records of the meeting.[23]

Saintgilligate would have been a street with work-places in or behind the houses where useful commodities could be bought. There were probably some shops or stalls (although none are mentioned in the surviving evidence), as well as storehouses for raw materials. The hospital staff must have come there to buy and order necessary items for themselves and their work: new habits for the brethren and almsmen made from locally-woven cloth (Thomas of Kyrkland, a tailor, lived beside the court-house in 1373/74); also boots (John Hextildesham, husband of Agnes, was a shoemaker before 1324); and articles fashioned from wood - furniture, kitchen utensils, agricultural implements and the like (Richard More was a carpenter during the mid- to late-fifteenth century). When all was ready the craftsmen or their apprentices would transport the hand-made articles to Kepier for approval and sale. A job well done would ensure another order.[24]

In spite of the hospital being on the periphery of the manor, the paths and roads to it were often busy ways. Staff and land-workers, burgesses supervising their affairs and relatives visiting elderly inmates would pass the time of day as they went about their business; or they might rub shoulders with pilgrims from distant parts of the country, who spoke their language with a different intonation that was sometimes hard to understand. The attraction of Kepier and the importance of Durham gave a variety to life on the hospital's estate that had not been experienced in the humble villages of Caldecotes and Clifton.

## 7. THE HOSPITAL OF ST MARY MAGDALEN[25]

Shortly after Puiset's time, Stephen the chaplain gave to the hospital of St Giles all his land called Southcroft, in the vicus of St Giles. This land became part of an exchange made in the first half of the thirteenth century. The hospital then ceded to the Prior and Convent 'twelve acres of land in our south croft below the vicus of St Giles towards the Wear', together with some of the land at Hurworth and Amerston, previously given by Gilbert Hansard. The document recording this is headed 'Hospital of St Mary Magdalen near Kepier'. Surtees, Barmby and M. Cornford (V.C.H. II) all thought that it referred to the origin of the smaller hospital.

Professor H.S. Offler, however, believed that a charter, not noticed by the other authors, told a different story. In it Bishop William of St Barbara (1143-52) makes known his grant of land in Sherburn 'to St Mary Magdalen and the sick people who dwell there'. This land can be identified with sixty acres 'in one large Close called Maudeleynleys before the Gate of Shirburn Hospital', which was mentioned in a pre- Dissolution list of the possessions

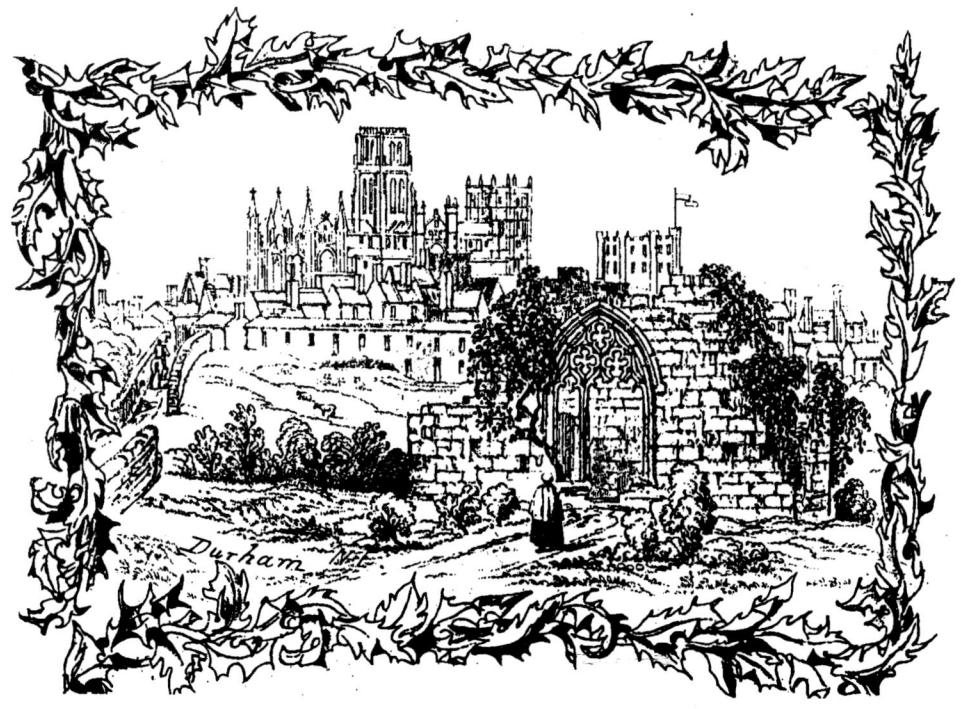

R. W. Billings

6. St Mary Magdalen Hospital, 1846.

of Magdalen Hospital. On the evidence of St Barbara's charter Offler considers that 'we seem entitled to set the foundation of St Mary Magdalen hospital off Gilesgate back before the middle of the twelfth century'. Possibly St Barbara founded Magdalen Hospital to take in some of the elderly victims of Cumin's misrule. (At that time the Hospital of St Giles was itself trying to recover from the attacks made on it and may have been unable to cope with its full complement of inmates.) In that case its work would have begun before the move of St Giles' Hospital to Kepier. This early date for Magdalen Hospital is supported by the fact that Godric's sister, Burcwen, retired from Finchale, where she had lived for a time, to an unnamed hospital. This is unlikely to have been that of St Giles, which had no woman member of staff to care for her. If Magdalen Hospital, which is known to have had women inmates in the fifteenth century, was in existence, it would have been able to receive the noted hermit's sister. Burcwen is recorded to have been buried in Durham and her grave was probably in the little hospital cemetery.[26]

After the 1180s Magdalen hospital would have been reduced in importance by the nearness of the wealthier establishment at Kepier, the lands of which surrounded it. Apparently the Cathedral Priory took over the lesser house and by the thirteenth century it was under the control of the monastic almoner. The master of the almonry school came to the hospital twice a week to say mass for the inmates (brethren and sisters). The chapel was rebuilt for a second time in the mid-fifteenth century. It was dedicated on 16 May 1451 by the suffragan bishop, with the assistance of John Lound, master of Kepier Hospital, and others.[27]

The land on which the hospital was built covered 24´ acres. It also constituted a parish. People living there (probably servants) worshipped at the chapel, which had full parochial status: a wedding is known to have taken place there in 1420-1, a marble stone was bought for the foot of the font in 1450-1 and a stranger, staying on the holding of Robert Johnson, within the parish, was buried 1515-6. Although it is first recorded in 1428-9 there is a strong probability that the little parish came into being before that of St Giles. It is most unlikely that, in the thirteenth century, by which time all parish boundaries were firmly drawn, the master of Kepier would meekly allow a sizeable area of his own parish to be removed (with its dues) in order to form a new one.[28]

## 8. WILLIAM WICKWANE, ARCHBISHOP OF YORK, AT KEPIER

In July 1283, after the death of Bishop Robert of Holy Island, the archbishop of York, William Wickwane, came to Durham. He was asserting his right as archbishop to visit the monastery while the see was vacant. The Prior and Convent, however, denied his metropolitan rights and refused him entrance. Angrily, he retired to St Nicholas' church in the market place, where he pronounced sentence of excommunication against the prior and obedientiaries (senior monks). This action aroused the youths of the town and they became so noisy and violent that the archbishop was frightened. Guided by Guichard de Charon and Peter de Thoresby (the late bishop's steward and treasurer, respectively), he fled down the steps at the side of the church 'towards the schools' and along the waterside to the safety of Kepier Hospital. In the uproar his palfrey had an ear cut off and, but for the intervention of the two officials, it was believed that the archbishop himself might have been killed.

## 9. THE BISHOPS AND KEPIER

### Antony Bek

Patrons often claimed free board and lodging at their hospitals for themselves and their retinues. Bishop Antony Bek (1283-1311) is known to have used Kepier in this way on two occasions. On 16 March 1289/90 Bek left Wark-on-Tweed, where he had been engaged in preliminary negotiations for a marriage between the new Scottish queen, Margaret, Maid of Norway, and Prince Edward of England. He reached Durham on 24 March and stayed the night at Kepier Hospital, doubtless keeping the Vigil of the Annunciation in the chapel there. The next morning he celebrated high mass in the cathedral before hurrying south to report to Edward I at Woodstock. Unfortunately, his diplomacy came to nothing when the Maid died later in the year.

In May 1300, during an escalating dispute with the Prior and Convent, Bek set up a blockade of the monastery to prevent anyone leaving to take appeals to York or Rome. This lasted into September. The priors of York and Whitby arrived inopportunely on 26 July to carry out the routine triennial visitation of the Benedictine houses in the province of York. They unwisely sympathised with the defiant monks and, as a result, on 27 July their servants and horses were seized by the bishop's men, who reported the matter to the bishop, then at Stockton. Bek was moved to great anger by all this and early the next morning he rode to Kepier and there held a meeting of his council to consider what should best be done.

On hearing that the bishop was at Kepier the prior of York came to him 'and deferentially and humbly asked that same father [i.e. Bek] whether, of his special grace, he would give permission for himself and his companion, that is, the prior of Whitby, and his household and his possessions, to go away.' After long deliberation this was allowed on condition that the visiting priors revoked any criticism they had made of those monks who were adherents of the bishop; also that they swore an oath on the Bible that they would do nothing further to the prejudice of the bishop. The two priors willingly satisfied these requirements, 'which having been done, they joyfully left Durham by the said father's special permission.'

### Letters dated at Kepier

Sometimes the bishops called at Kepier and, while they were there, conducted certain secretarial business. A copy of a letter of Antony Bek's survives, dated at the hospital on 23 February 1310/11, and there are copies of fourteen letters of Richard Kellaw (1311-16), his successor, all dated at Kepier between March 1311/12 and November 1314. It is likely that Kellaw and members of his staff stayed overnight, now and then, for some of these letters were written on consecutive dates, two in March 1311/12 and three in November 1314.[29] Other bishops probably treated the hospital in the same way.

### Ordinations

Ordinations to any of the four minor and three major orders of ministry took place generally in the cathedral, the chapels of the episcopal castles and manors and in some parish churches. There was one occasion in 1342 when the chapel at Kepier was the setting for such a service. It occurred on Sunday 22 September when nineteen men received the first tonsure (i.e. the shaving of the crown of the head) as doorkeepers. They were admitted to this lowest of the minor orders by Richard, Bishop of Bisaccia, Bishop Bury's suffragan, on the authority of the diocesan.[30]

All these comings and goings must have brought excitement into the monotonous lives of the hospital inmates. In fact, such visits were to their detriment, for the endowments that had been made for the care of the poor were being expended on people who had other means of support.

## 10. A CORRODIAN

Patrons made use of their hospitals as places of retirement for their old servants, granting them a corrody (i.e. provision for maintenance), which was paid by the hospital. Bishop Kellaw sent William of Pencher to Kepier 'on account of his faithful service'. There he was given a robe 'of the kind of our servants' (presumably the special habit worn by the brethren) and an annuity of 6s. 8d. - enough to buy him 'all other necessities'. While he remained in good health he was to have his meals in the hall at the same table as the brethren. If he became poorly and unable to get about he was to be looked after and given whatever he needed. This is the only mention of a corrodian at Kepier, but it is likely that there were others who benefited from a bishop's generosity, although this would have been at the expense of the hospital.

## 11. THE SCOTTISH WAR

### King Edward I

The events following the death of the Maid of Norway led to Edward I's invasion of Scotland in March 1295/96, and the protracted Scottish war, in which Kepier suffered along with the rest of the north of England. Having conquered the defiant kingdom, Edward returned to the south but travelled back again in 1298 to quell a rising against the occupation forces. On his way to the border he stopped at Kepier hospital for the night of 17 June. Antony Bek was at the manor of Bishop Auckland on that date but may have come to Durham later in the day or early the next morning. King and bishop probably left Durham together on 18 June, were in Alnwick on 26 June, joined the main body of troops at Roxburgh and defeated the Scots at the battle of Falkirk on 22 July. Not until sixteen years later did the Scots dare to challenge the English to another full-scale pitched battle.

## Queen Isabella

After the death of Edward I at Burgh-on-Sands, Cumberland, in 1307, his son, Edward II, retired to England. During the following three years the unyielding Scots, under Robert Bruce, strengthened their position and consolidated their gains. The failure of the invaders to control the situation demanded the presence of the king. Edward II rode to Berwick in 1310 accompanied by the sixteen-years-old Queen Isabella. From there he conducted an unsuccessful campaign in southern Scotland between September 1310 and August 1311. The queen left Berwick in the spring and reached Kepier on 21 April, where she and her attendants stayed the night. They continued on their journey the following day, the master being paid £18 17s. 9d. for their expenses.

Kepier was perhaps suggested as a suitable place to receive the queen because women were not welcome close to St Cuthbert's shrine (the saint being thought to have an aversion to them). For this reason, twenty-two years later, Isabella's daughter-in-law, Queen Philippa, was obliged to move from the prior's house (in the cathedral precincts) to the castle, in the middle of the night.

For the old men who had come to Kepier to end their lives in quietness the presence of these two exalted personages was almost beyond belief. The sight of the warrior king and the young queen-consort, the bustle of their attendants, the clattering of the horses' hooves, the scurrying about of servants, the gleaning of news and gossip, even some small assistance rendered by the more able-bodied among themselves, were experiences they would gladly recall for future inmates and would remember for the remainder of their days.

## A fire at Kepier

Between the two royal visits a part of the hospital buildings was destroyed. On 17 May 1306 a fire broke out in the muniment room and all the charters and other records of the house were destroyed. This was a serious loss as, without them, there was no legal proof of what lands and endowments the hospital possessed. Bishop Kellaw appointed a commission on 6 December 1311 to enquire into these matters. Counterparts of some of the charters were in existence and others were verified on oath. New copies of all the documents were confirmed by Kellaw on 11 March 1311/2.

Surtees says that Kellaw's commission was directed to investigate the 'damage perpetrated in the hospital of Kepier by the Scots'. Neither of the surviving copies nor Kellaw's confirmation of the charters, while mentioning the fire, name the Scots as its cause. In any case, there was no Scottish invasion in 1306. After 1311 the north was constantly harried by the Scots. In 1312 the town of Durham itself was attacked and set on fire and, before June 1315, goods (unspecified) belonging to the hospital were seized. Later, these circumstances may have led to the Kepier fire of 1306 being mistakenly attributed also to the Scots. Possibly the copy of the commission that Surtees saw was kept with a note to that effect.

## The depressed state of the hospital, 1312

The object of Bruce's raids of 1312 was to obtain money, cattle and corn: where an estate paid for immunity it was left alone; where it did not it was systematically plundered. It seems probable that some of the lands belonging to Kepier suffered in this incursion and that the hospital lost a large proportion of its tithes and gillycorn. Bishop Kellaw, concerned about the 'depressed state' of the hospital, made fresh endowments to enable it to continue and multiply its charitable works. In July 1312 he granted the tithes of all assarts near Gateshead and at Brounsyde (in the parish of Auckland), until he should order otherwise concerning them. This extra income was also meant to provide two chaplains in addition to those already ministering.

### Disagreement about certain tithes, 1314

Most parishes in Durham and Northumberland suffered from the inroads made by the Scots, and rectors resented seeing any part of the remaining crops (thought to be tithes owing to them) going to some distant religious house. Two known cases were about the garb tithes due to the masters and brethren of Kepier. These were the garbs (or sheaves) which were part of Flambard's endowment.

The problem was only dealt with by the intervention of Bishop Kellaw. He settled matters between the master and brethren and the rectors involved, Thomas de Goldesburgh, rector of Easington, also archdeacon of Durham, and Thomas de Hessewell, rector of Sedgefield (and Kellaw's cousin), by two deeds of arbitration, dated 22 and 23 April 1314, respectively. Firstly, he decided that the Easington tithes, which the hospital had received 'time out of mind', should continue to be paid without hindrance. Furthermore, he declared that the master and brethren should celebrate a mass yearly in the church at Kepier on the anniversary of Bishop Antony Bek (3 March). This would have pleased Thomas of Goldesburgh who had been appointed archdeacon by Bek; he was the bishop's nephew and one of the executors of his will. Secondly, concerning the tithes of Hardwick (which had been granted by the then bishop of Durham 'some time ago', in exchange for those of Sedgefield), they were to be sent to the hospital, as in the past, but the master and brethren were to pay the rector of Sedgefield 20s. annually. The rector was obliged to go to Kepier for his payment on the feast of St John the Baptist (24 June).[31]

### Depredation by the Scots, 1315

After the Scottish victory at the battle of Bannockburn in June 1314 there were regular and frequent attacks on northern England, during which the estates of the hospital were despoiled. Bishop Kellaw, in expressing his concern about this, gave a brief description of the services provided at Kepier: 'divine worship, hospitality to those arriving, support and recreation of the needy, and other works and burdens of charity in the said hospital, where a multitude of the poor converge to beg for sustenance. . . .' Because of its 'evident and notorious poverty' it now needed 'succour . . . from another source. . . .' This help Kellaw proceeded to give: on 1 June 1315 he created a fourteenth prebend in the collegiate church of St Andrew Auckland. This office was to be appropriated forever to the master of Kepier, who would have a stall in the choir and receive the tithes from associated lands. The duties of the prebendary were to be performed by a sub-deacon, with a stipend of thirty shillings a year.

The master was required also to appoint two more chaplains at Kepier (making seven priests there altogether, excluding the master) to celebrate for the bishop himself, his predecessors and successors. The fact that the new total number of chaplains was only seven shows that the hospital had not been able to support its original staff of six, let alone those endowed later. Possibly the two mentioned by Kellaw three years earlier had not been engaged and therefore he was repeating the directions about them.

The number of casuals being assisted every evening by distributions of food was to be increased by ten people. This is the first record of out-door relief at Kepier, but it may have been customary from the beginning.

On the anniversary of the bishop's death one of the priests was to celebrate mass for his soul. Then provision was made for a commemorative feast: thirteen poor people, presumably the permanent inmates, were each to receive bread, pottage, drink and three herrings. The bishop died the following year on 9 October so, from 1316 onwards, that day was kept at Kepier as a religious and secular festival, something akin to Christmas and Easter. For seven days afterwards the other priests, in turn, said further masses for the bishop's soul.

The master's involvement in more pressing occupations was acknowledged by exempting him from being present at synods, chapter-meetings, visitations and convocations.[32] It was expected that he would often be away in attendance on the bishop but, apart from such times, he was to be resident in the hospital.

The fact that a sub-deacon could be placed at Auckland and two chaplains at Kepier, and that the issue of food to the poor could be increased out of the new grant of tithes demonstrates the great value of Kellaw's donation.

The Auckland settlement was only part of the aid given by Kellaw. In a deed dated the very next day he first praised the hospital for its charitable works, but regretted that it had been 'reduced to great poverty and want'. He blamed this on 'the invasion of the Scots, who were not afraid to extend their thieving hands to the hospital's property.' As a result 'it [could not], of itself, rise again unless there [was] someone to raise it up and, when re-established, support it with abundant generous help.' Kellaw then confirmed the grant of the tithes of the assarts of Gateshead, which had been made as a temporary measure in 1312.[33]

The deprived condition described in this deed shows that, although the ownership of land and its produce had made the institution wealthy, such wealth could easily be lost through the action of marauders. Not until Edward III's victory at the battle of Halidon Hill in July 1333 was the constant threat of Scottish raids removed.

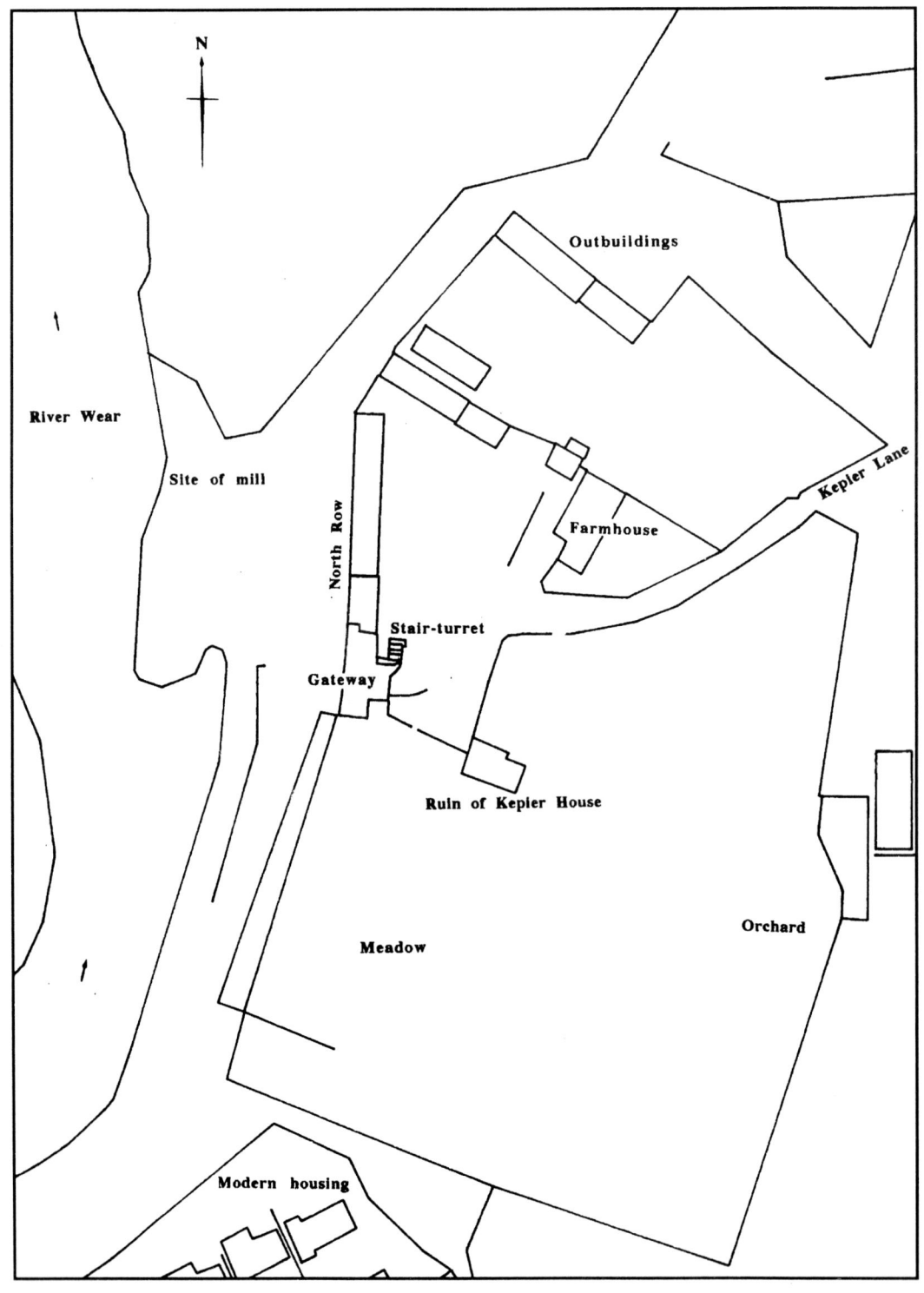

7. Plan of Kepier Farm site.

## 12. THE BUILDINGS AT KEPIER[34]

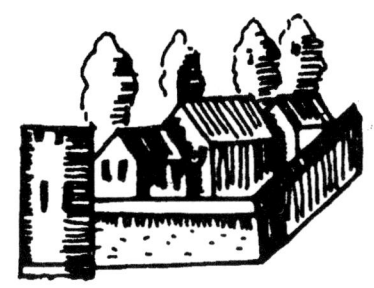

The end of the Scottish wars brought a period of respite and led to a major rebuilding programme at Kepier. Both the bishop and the master were aware that the Scots might descend on Durham again so it was built for strength and security. Again, stone from Kepier quarry would have been used and, in view of the amount needed, perhaps also from Frankland quarry on the other side of the river. Some small idea of the hospital's appearance at this time may be gained from the surviving buildings, helped by the simplified sketch on Christopher Schwyzer's map of Durham, 1595, and the three drawings by S.H. Grimm (dated 1777-84). Much has been dismantled, altered or put to other uses since the Middle Ages, so certain suggestions are purely conjectural.

*Martin Roberts*
8. Kepier Hospital, from Christopher Schwyzer's map, 1595.

Bishop Richard of Bury (1333-45) built the impressive gatehouse, with its attractive ornamentation. Above the outside (west front) of the gateway, high up on the wall, are two

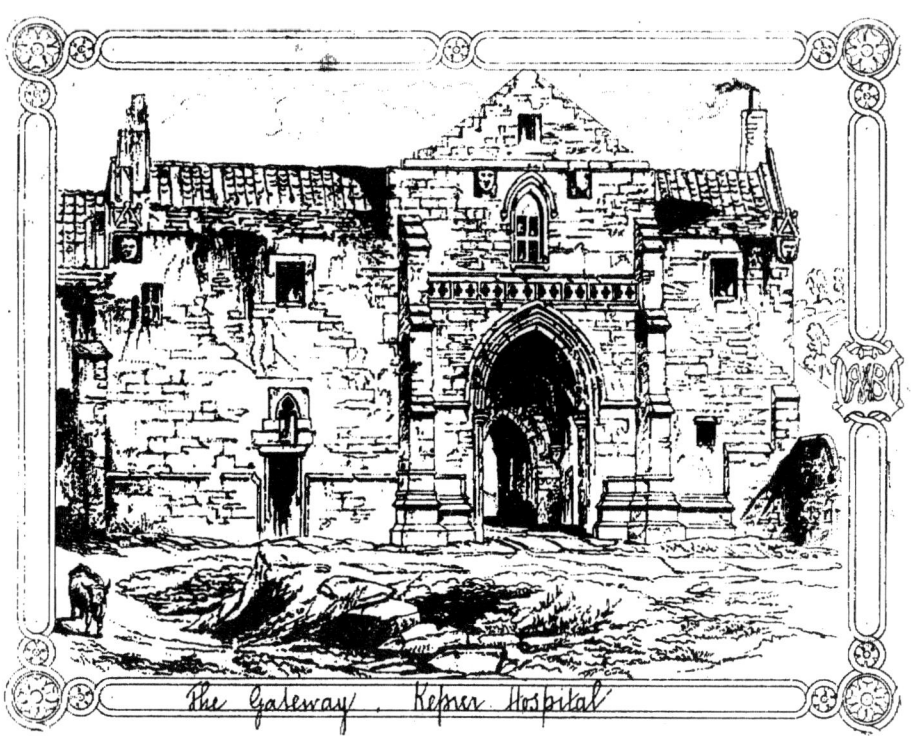

*R. W. Billings*
9. Kepier Gateway, west face, 1846.

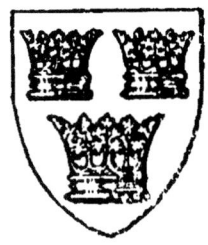 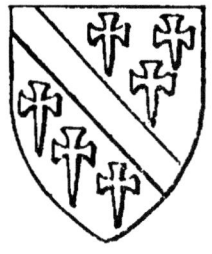

*C. H. Hunter Blair*
10. Kepier Gateway, shields on west front.

shields, both decayed. It has been suggested that the one on the left - azure three crowns or - attributed to St Edmund, was here used by Bury as his personal heraldic device, although the shield of the Suffolk saint usually had an arrow through or between the crowns. The one on the right is that of Edmund Howard - gules crusilly fitchy and a bend argent - who occurs as master from 1341-5. Immediately over the arch is a line of quatrefoils, a pleasing feature clearly seen by R.W. Billings in 1846, now much eroded. The gateway is vaulted in two bays, with cross ribs meeting in carved bosses which Boyle, writing in 1892, described as 'beautiful', although their condition has deteriorated. Just inside the outer arch there are two interesting but crumbling corbels, the one on the north side being carved as a small frog-like creature and the one on the south as a crab.

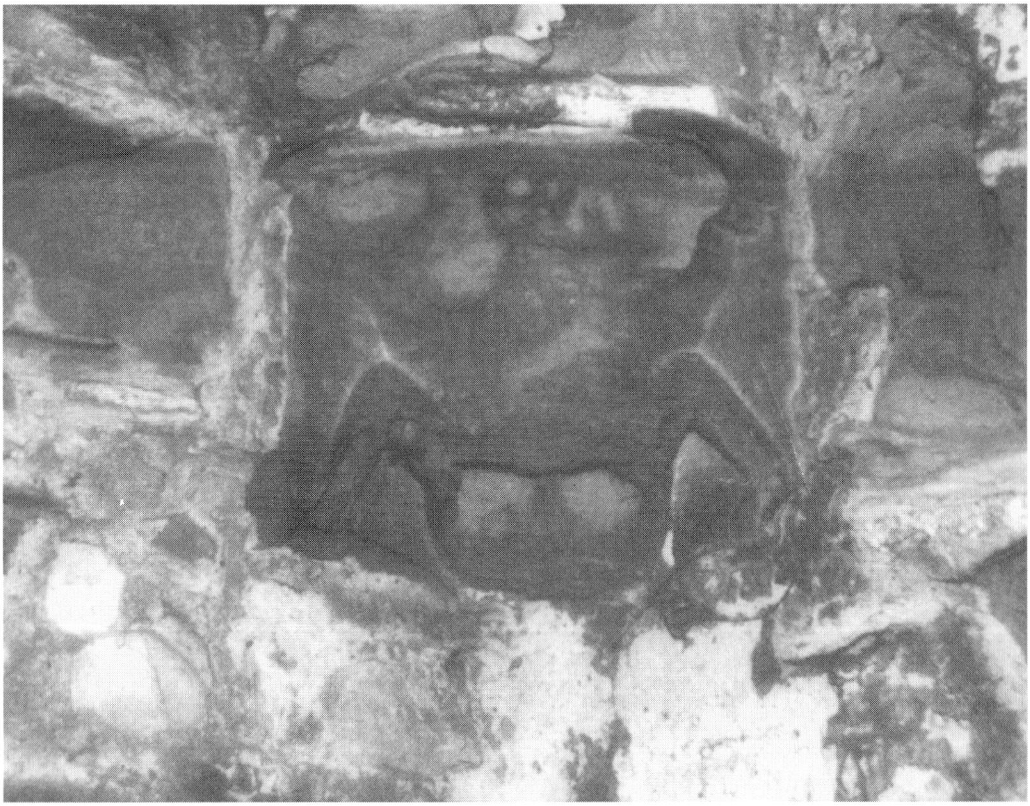

*M. F. Richardson*
11. Kepier Gateway, carved corbel showing a crablike creature.

Boyle also noticed staples of door hinges in the walls (only one remains) showing that there had been two sets of doors, at the outer and middle arches, respectively. These would have been attended to by porters whose rooms, the northernmost of which has a wide fireplace, flank the entrance. On the inner (east) side a newel staircase (now blocked) led to the upper floor. This is still inhabited and reached by an external stone stairway of later date.

Early in 1994 the roofs of the gatehouse - central, north wing and south wing - were recovered. This presented an opportunity to investigate the roof structure. There is evidence for an early roof although many of the timbers have been re-used at least once during succeeding centuries. The wing roofs are now of a slightly lower pitch than the medieval originals and this has caused some alteration in the gables. The whole of the roof-area is covered in red clay pantiles, but was formerly roofed in stone.

The gateway faces west onto the riverside and the road from Durham runs through it to a courtyard approximately rectangular in shape. On the opposite side is another fourteenth-century building, on twelfth-century foundations, now a farmhouse. Its former use is not known, but there is part of an original fireplace in the main ground-floor room. The lane beside it led to the hospital's two granges. It is possible that there was a second sturdy, but less pretentious, gate at the junction of this lane with the courtyard.

A range of buildings, with fine late medieval roofing, dated shortly after 1552 (by tree-

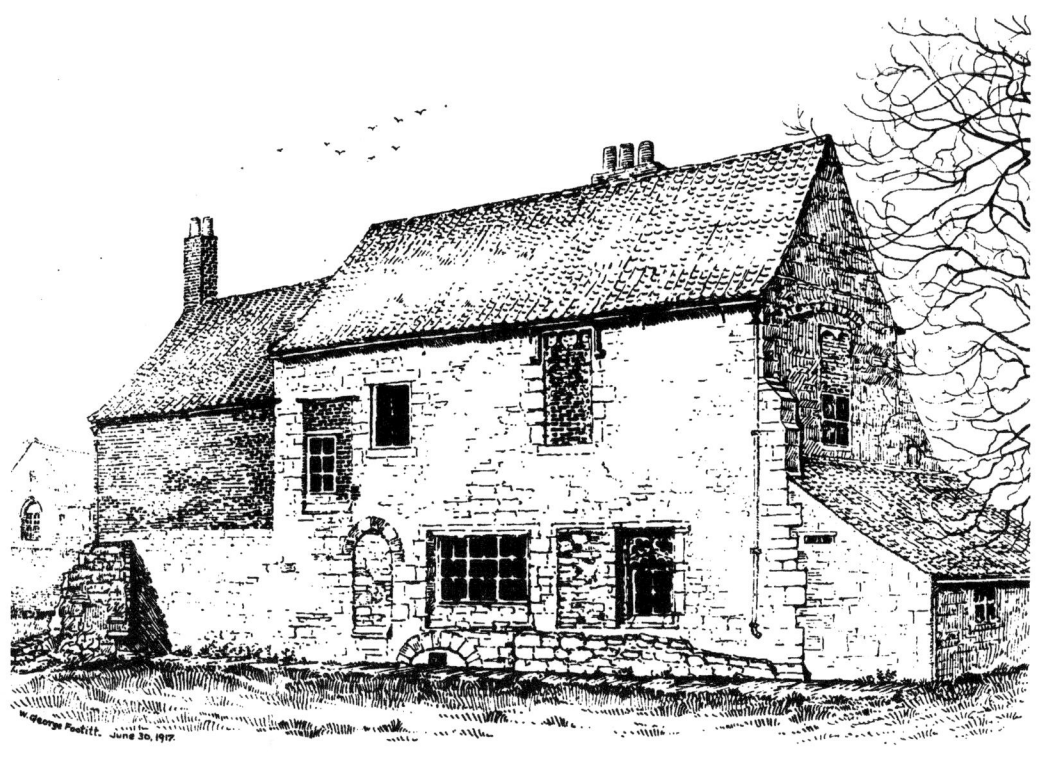

*W. G. Footitt*

12. Kepier Farmhouse, facing east (*see also* 30a and 30b on page 56).

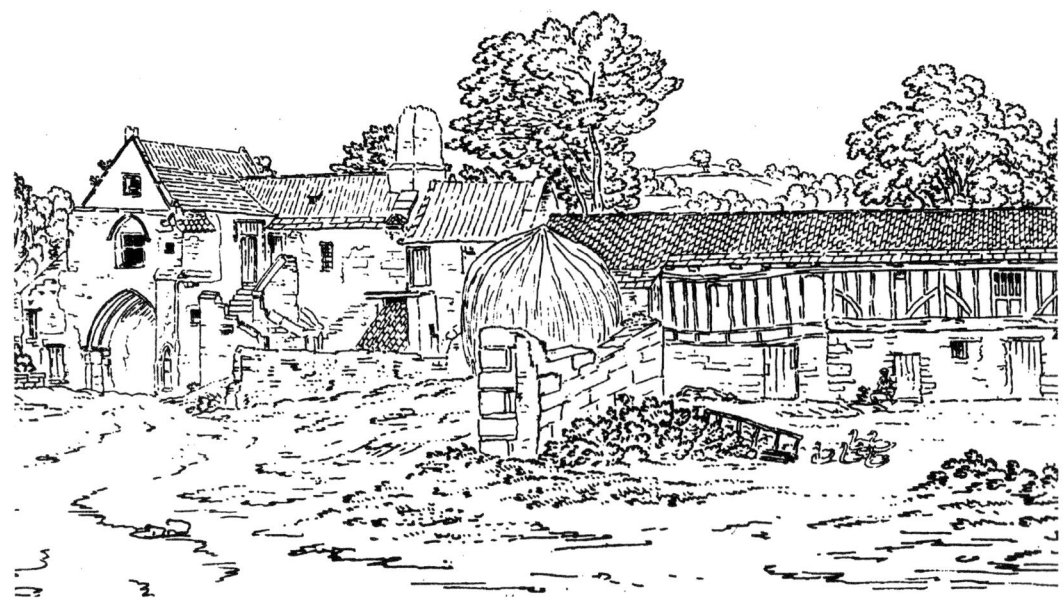

*S.H. Grimm*

13. Kepier Gateway: east face

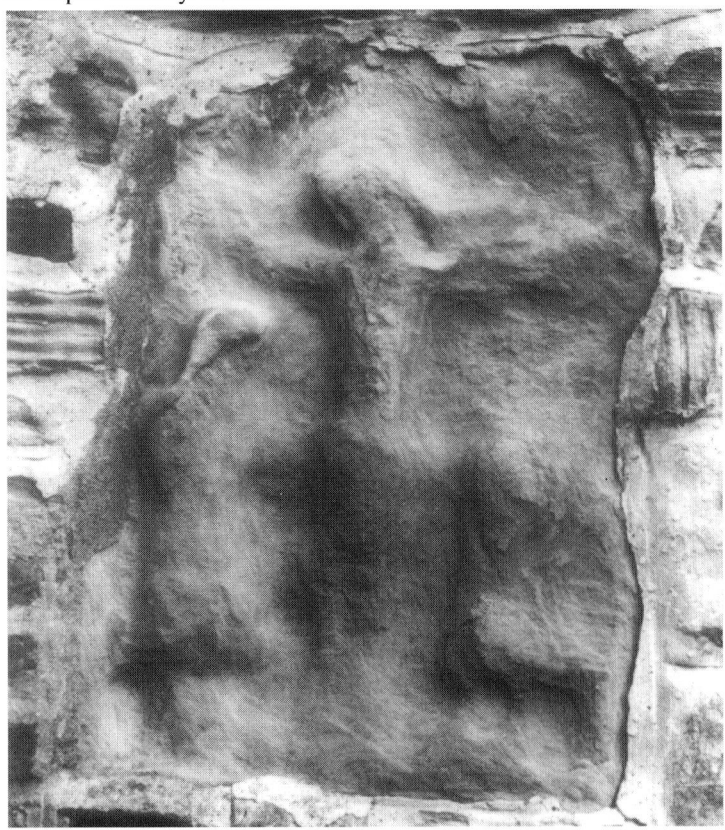

*M.F. Richardson*

14. Kepier Farmhouse: sculptured crucifixion, perhaps from the chapel. The figures of Mary and John flank the cross but the whole is much weathered.

ring dating) extends north from the gatehouse. The drawings of S.H. Grimm show the upper storey to be timber-framed, and this construction is still visible on the inside. It appears to be of the same construction as the roof and so is of the same date. Vestiges of it can be seen externally on the east side, although largely encased in stone-work. The row is unlikely to have been used for human accommodation as it is completely open to the roof with no evidence of sub-division, its tie-beams are too low for moving about easily, there are no windows on the river side and no fire- places, which might have been expected at this date. It seems, therefore, to have been some sort of service building, replacing or modernising an earlier construction.

The chapel would have occupied a prominent position. On Christopher Schwyzer's plan of Durham, 1595, the simple drawing of the hospital shows a west tower on the south side of the courtyard. It is reminiscent of the chapel at Sherburn Hospital and may well have represented the position of the former chapel of Kepier. This idea is supported by the fact that some 14th-century burials were found north- east of its site in 1961, suggesting that this was part of the churchyard adjacent to the chapel. A much-weathered stone carving of the Crucifixion, flanked by St Mary and St John, now built into the west wall of the farmhouse, almost certainly belonged in the chapel originally. A carved stone head of a 15th-century gentleman, also found in 1961, was perhaps a corbel, put in to honour a generous donor.

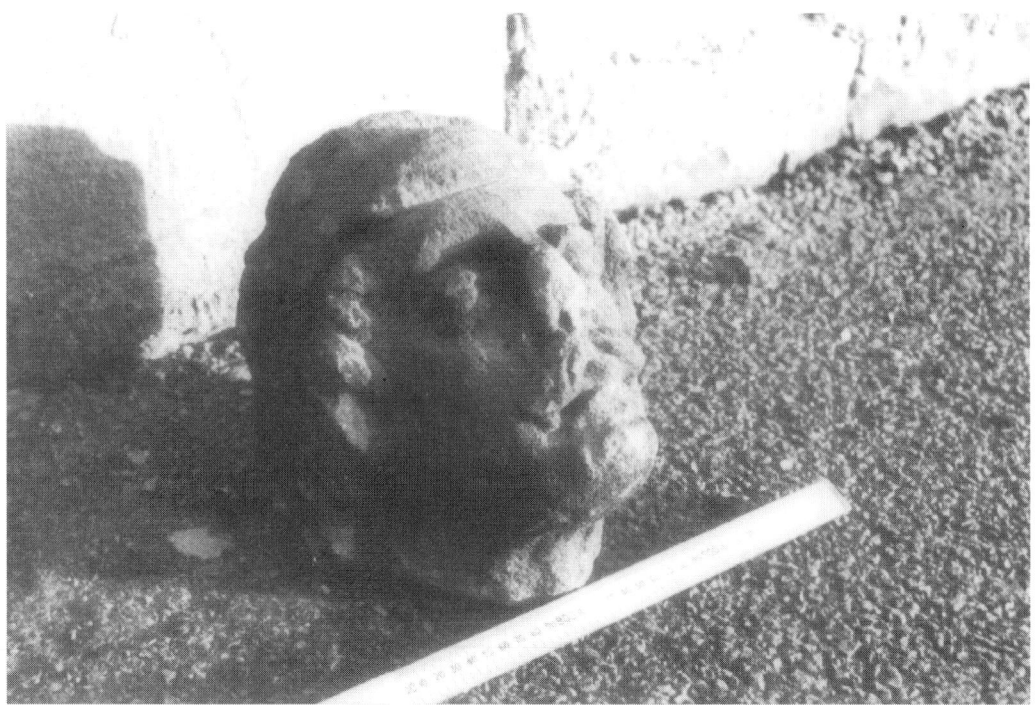

M. F. Richardson

15. Carved head (corbel ?) 15th century layman, perhaps a wealthy donor; discovered buried in the orchard in 1961.

The whole complex was probably on the near-quadrangular plan often associated with medieval hospitals and colleges, buildings on the four sides of the courtyard forming a compact enclosure. When the gates were locked at night the community, with its guests, was safe from unwelcome intruders. The master must have felt justified in the expense of the re-building when the Scots invaded the north of England yet again in October 1346. Then the whole of Durham was in danger until they were defeated at the battle of Neville's Cross, on the western side of the city.

## 13. THE BLACK DEATH

In 1349 the Black Death, which had reached the south of England in the previous summer, swept across Durham and Northumberland. Along with everyone else, the tenants of the widespread lands of the hospital were affected and many of them died. The crops failed because there were few men left to harvest them or to sow the land again. The effects of this desolation continued to be felt in the succeeding years, when Kepier had to endure the loss of some tithes and thraves. The house was reduced to great poverty and in 1353 steps were taken to mitigate this. It obtained the advowson and glebe of Hunstanworth in an exchange with the Prior and Convent for an annual out-rent of 13s. 4d. from the grange of Caldecotes. This concluded unsatisfactory negotiations begun in 1331. Even in 1353 the settlement was something of a mixed blessing for the hospital: the chancel and the rectory house were both in need of repair and it proved difficult to find a priest willing to serve there; also, the revenues were diminished, doubtless because the village itself had not escaped the plague.[35]

The following year a murrain (perhaps foot-and-mouth disease) afflicted the hospital's sheep and 600 of them died. Because of the prolonged deprivation Bishop Hatfield (1345-81), in 1355, granted an indulgence of 40 days (to which could be added 300 days already given by his predecessors) for all those who contributed to the relief of the poverty-stricken institution. The rectors and parochial chaplains of the diocese were commanded by the bishop to promote the matter in their churches. They were to 'clearly expound the same in the spirit of charity' and to send any money collected to the master and brethren without delay. This measure was not unlike a modern charity appeal, and was a recognised form of fund-raising. In return for a donation the giver was remitted some of the penance awaiting him in purgatory.

## 14. POOR SCHOLARS

When Robert Wyclif, master of Kepier, died in 1423 he left two shillings 'to each poor scholar sitting at the skepham within the hall of the aforesaid hospital'. This money would have made life a little easier for the scholars who might have bought, for instance, a supply of parchment, some candles and a pair of gloves with it. The skepham was perhaps a basket from which the youths received a dole of food.

There is no other mention of scholars at Kepier, but it will be remembered that, when Archbishop Wickwane was hurrying there from St Nicholas' church in 1283, he fled 'towards the schools'. If these were still in existence in 1423 pupils from them may have been provided with a daily meal at the hospital. However, the early 'schools' are not heard of again after 1283, so it is possible that Kepier's poor scholars attended another seat of learning in the city.

The presence of lively lads would have been a mixed blessing to the aged residents. Doubtless one of the staff was given the responsibility for seeing that they behaved themselves and were not too noisy or active.

## 15. ST NICHOLAS' CHURCH AND OLD DURHAM

The payment of thraves was a great burden to the peasants, who must have put obstacles in the way of sending them to Kepier whenever they could. As a result the revenues of the hospital had fallen considerably by the middle of the fifteenth century. They were then not sufficient 'for the maintenance, building and repair of the houses, and keeping hospitality for which it was chiefly founded'.

In an effort to put the hospital on a more secure economic footing, the master, John Lound, appealed to Bishop Robert Neville (1437-57) for help in 1443. His petition for the appropriation of St Nicholas' church, Durham, to the hospital was granted and nothing more is heard of any financial embarrassment. As at Hunstanworth, the hospital became the rector, putting in a vicar at a small stipend, receiving the larger share of the parish income and becoming the owner of the glebe (i.e. the land for the support of the parson).

The glebe of St Nicholas' was the manor of Old Durham, which was adjacent to the southern boundary of the hospital's Durham city lands and close to the river Wear as it approached the peninsula. In 1479 this property was leased by Ralph Booth, then master of Kepier, to his brother, Richard Booth, and his descendants, for 99 years.

## 16. BOARD AND LODGING AT KEPIER

The pilgrims' guest-house cannot have been used to full capacity in winter and during certain seasons of the farming year. Because of this the hospital would sometimes have vacant accommodation which it could let as a means of supplementing its income.

At some time between 29 September 1475 and 15 August 1476 the bishop's Durham mills were overhauled. Major work was done on them and on the dams, the necessary wood being obtained from the woods of Frankland on the north bank of the Wear. Many carpenters and labourers were employed and they were lodged at Kepier Hospital, receiving breakfast and an evening meal. They stayed there for two or three months, 'during the time that the mills were being repaired'. The steward of Kepier was paid £37 for their maintenance, a considerable sum indicative of a large work-force. The carpenters and labourers may have worked on the mills from October to December, if the weather was good, or after 20 March, when the pilgrims who came for St Cuthbert's day had gone home. One can only wonder about the feelings of the inmates towards a crowd of noisy men coming back to the hospital precincts every night.[36]

## 17. THE MASTERS OF KEPIER

In Bishop Hugh of Le Puiset's original rules the head of the hospital is called 'the master'. This remained the usual title, but there were variations in certain documents. 'Master or custodian' was quite common, and 'governor', also 'rector', occurred at times.[37]

The masters of Kepier were usually senior executives of the bishops, for whom the hospital post meant an addition to their incomes. Peter de Thoresby, for instance, was Antony Bek's chancellor, one of his justices and receiver-general; Robert Wyclif was appointed chancellor, receiver-general and constable of Durham castle by Bishop Skirlaw (1388-1406); and William Franklyn was chancellor and receiver-general to Bishops Ruthall (1509-23) and Wolsey (1523-9).

Many of these men held benefices also, from which they drew the fruits of office but put in a parochial chaplain to do the parish work. William Legat, master in 1348 until his death in 1362, was rector of Brancepeth at the same time;[38] and Hugh Herle, who had been master since 1381, was collated to the rectory of Easington in 1388, keeping both positions until he died five years later.[39] They may have visited their rectories at times - it seems that Robert Wyclif stayed occasionally at Rudby (of which he was rector from 1377 to his death in 1423), for his roll of legacies mentions several bed-hangings there, including a set with the arms of his family embroidered on it.[40]

A master of Kepier was a man of standing in the city and beyond. He gained a home - a suite of rooms for his personal use (fit to receive royalty, on occasion), stabling, servants, a supply of good food - which was conveniently near the diocesan capital. When governmental work took him far afield this riverside retreat awaited his return. There he could enjoy some leisure and see to the business of the hospital before leaving orders to a deputy and returning to attendance on the bishop.

Masters appointed for their own benefit, rather than that of the hospital, were not always ideally suited to the task. They were often absent on the bishop's business and so might prove careless administrators of the hospital's resources. Patrons were supposed to make a yearly inspection of the premises and to check the accounts and inventory. The bishops of Durham seem to have done this rarely and then only when they suspected that all was not well or if rumours of mismanagement had reached them. Bishop Richard Kellaw summoned Peter de Thoresby (who had been appointed by his predecessor, Antony Bek) to appear in the hospital chapel on Sunday 27 June 1311 to answer a charge of misappropriating the goods of the house. As one of Bek's leading officers he must have been a master who neglected the duties but absorbed the profits of the post. Kellaw's initial enquiry led to a full-scale visitation of the hospital for 'the reforming and correcting of defects and corrupt excesses' there. As a result Thoresby must have been dismissed, for Hugh de Monte Alto is named as master in a charter dated 24 December. Kellaw probably had

Thoresby's shortcomings in mind when, in creating the new prebend at Auckland, he specified that the master must always reside in the hospital unless he was accompanying the bishop.

Hugh de Monte Alto (or Mohaut), whose name was probably a Latinised form of an English surname like 'Hill' or 'High-hill', had been a monk of the cathedral priory when Kellaw was the sub-prior. Even a master of Kepier was not entirely secure for he was dependent on his bishop's favour. Mohaut was made aware of this three weeks after the death of Kellaw. On Sunday 31 October Simon de Eycote, of the king's household, came to Kepier and claimed, rightly, that King Edward II had appointed him to be master of the hospital. Mohaut objected to this claim but Eycote 'ejected him from the hospital by force and wasted his goods'. Mohaut appealed to the king for restitution but to no avail. Eycote remained for four years until 22 November 1320 when Mohaut was reinstated. The returned master and the brethren granted Eycote £10 worth of land in Amerston, Hurworth and elsewhere. This displaced master is last heard of in 1323 as King's Clerk in the Marshalsea.[41]

A conscientious master with a sense of responsibility would be able to give satisfactory supervision in spite of frequent absences. This is borne out by the result of a visitation ordered by Bishop Thomas Langley in 1437. At that time the master was Richard Buckley, who had been the bishop's receiver-general since 1422. His task of collecting the revenues took him out of the hospital on numerous occasions and he had apparently been accused of maladministration of the goods of the house. After a searching inquiry had taken place and the accounts had been audited he was given a full acquittal for his conduct of the hospital's affairs (25 August). So much confidence was placed in him that his office was granted to him for life. The bishop died on 20 November of that same year and Buckley was one of the executors of the will, by which he received £10 as a bequest. Two years later, in October 1439, Buckley resigned because of age and infirmity. Before appointing his successor, Bishop Robert Neville (1437-57) called for the hospital accounts to be brought to the treasury at Durham, where they were inspected and approved. He then granted the old man an annual pension of 40 marks (£26.66) out of the revenues of the hospital. This large amount was considered suitable for one who had served the bishopric well for 32 years. With it the former master could pass the remainder of his days (probably at Kepier) wanting for nothing. At the same time his pension was an additional expense for the hospital and it had to be paid till he died in 1446.[42]

Buckley was succeeded by John Lound, canon of Salisbury and holder of two rectories. It would seem that he was brought to Kepier by Bishop Robert Neville, who had been translated from Salisbury to Durham in 1437. Of noble, although illegitimate birth, his progress through the ranks of the Church owed much to family influence. (His illegitimacy was a bar to taking holy orders but this was overcome by payment for a papal dispensation.) Whilst master of Kepier he became also canon and prebendary of Howden, Yorkshire, in 1448, and chancellor to Bishop Neville in 1457 (being one of the supervisors of the bishop's will in that same year). He continued as chancellor, in certain years, to Bishop Booth. With income from all of these sources and probably with some means provided by his family as well, Lound was a wealthy man with a lot of money to invest.

By 1452 he had acquired a messuage and three tenements with gardens in the Bailey (on the site now covered by numbers 3 to 5 South Bailey) which he let to various tenants. This property, together called his 'mansion in the South Bailey', passed to the cathedral priory on his death in 1467. It was still being called 'Lound House' in 1541.

The last visitation was that of Bishop Cuthbert Tunstal (1530-59) in 1532. He informed the master, William Franklyn, that either he or his representatives would visit the hospital on 18 July because he had heard reports that the property had been wasted. The charters, inventory and accounts were to be exhibited in the chapel. There are no returns of this visitation but the master retained his position.[43]

Because the masters were personages of substance with more than one source of income they were able to live in comfort, even luxury. The will (dated at Kepier 8 September 1423) and inventory of Robert Wyclif show him to have been a very wealthy man, leaving generous amounts of money and silver-ware to churches and close associates; and several sets of bed-curtains and coverlets to friends. He left the hospital a cup with a perforated cover, a collection of 12 spoons and five books (two or these were for the personal use of John Middleton, one of the chaplains, during his lifetime). From his private rooms at Kepier he gave a set of red bed-hangings, with certain embroideries, to Robert Topping, and a red coverlet with the arms of Bishop Skirlaw on it to William Semar. (This last was probably bought from Skirlaw's goods, for which purchase the bishop gave permission in his will of 1406, Wyclif being one of the executors.) Each of the chaplains and each of the brethren received 6s 8d, a useful sum - the same as that paid annually to professional choirmasters when employed at the cathedral priory. This bequest distinguishes between the chaplains whose duties were mainly religious and the other members of staff who saw to the practicalities of running the household and the estates. It also shows that they were no longer bound by the vows of poverty which had been a requirement of the original rules.[44]

Ralph Booth was a nephew of Laurence Booth, Bishop of Durham (1457-76) and Archbishop of York (1476-80). Already canon and prebendary of Norton, rector of Longnewton and archdeacon of York, the mastership of Kepier came his way in 1479. In spite of these appointments, all of which he held till death, Bishop John Sherwood (1484-94) made him his chancellor in 1491, a position he continued to hold under Bishop Fox (1494-1501). He was thus for many years a prominent figure in the diocese. Towards the end of an energetic life he retired to Kepier and in February 1496/7 he lay on his deathbed. One of his last acts was to give into the hands of Thomas Swalwell, the monastic chancellor, two silver seals of office which he had used during the time of Bishop Sherwood. After the death of the bishop they were no longer needed and he had kept them at Kepier. Now he asked that they should be offered at the shrine of St Cuthbert, 'according to custom'. He further requested that five paternosters with the angelic salutation should be said for his late benefactor and for himself at the time of the offering. Swalwell performed this last duty on 5 February. Booth died a short time later and, presumably, was buried at Kepier, either in the chapel or in the graveyard attached to it.[45]

Not every master stayed at Kepier for life. Henry Gillow, who preceded Booth, resigned in 1479 in order to move to York as sub-dean.[46] Roger Layborn was the holder of several rectories in the Durham diocese - Longnewton, Sedgefield, Easington - and was also Archdeacon of Durham, when he became Master of Kepier in 1500. Three years later he left the diocese on elevation to the bishopric of Carlisle.[47]

In many ways the old men at Kepier must have felt like humble dependents in the home of a great lord. They would be aware of the master's arrivals and departures, of the wealth of his equipage, of his hastening messengers, of his presence at certain meals in the hall (even of his absence when he ate in private) and of his celebrating mass on special church festivals. They may have wondered, from time to time, about the differences between their own lowly lives and those of the masters, who gave priority to the demands of the posts they held at diocesan level and treated the inmates' needs as of secondary importance.

## MASTERS OF KEPIER HOSPITAL[48]

>
> Meldred, priest of St Giles', 1131
> Adam, occurs 1189
> Ralph, occ. between 1228 and 1237
> De Argentino, occ. between 1241 and 1249
> John de London, occ. 1254 and 1258
> Peter de Thoresby, 1291-1311
> Hugh de Monte Alto (alias Mohaut), 1311-16
> Simon de Eycote, appointed 17 October 1316, ejected 1320
> Hugh de Monte Alto, reinstated 22 November, 1320-40
> Edmund Howard, occ. 1341-5
> William Legat, 1348-62
> Richard Roter, app. 14 January 1363
> Hugh Herle, app. 26 July 1381; occ. 1388
> Robert Wyclif, occ. before 1405 - till death, 1423
> Richard Buckley, app. 1423; resigned 1439
> John Lound, app. 1439; occ. 1457
> Henry Gillow, occ. 1465-79
> Ralph Booth, app. 1479-97
> Thomas Colston, app. 20 April 1497 - 1499/1500
> Roger Layborn, 1499/1500-1503
> Thomas Wytton, 1503
> John Boer, 1504-15
> William Franklyn, 1515-45

## 18. THE HOSPITAL IN 1535

A good deal of information about hospitals in 1535 is contained in the Valor Ecclesiasticus, Henry VIII's survey of ecclesiastical incomes. It was compiled by commissions in the different bishoprics, William Franklyn being a member of that for Durham.

Bishop Tunstal sent off the Durham returns on 21 July.[49]

Kepier was then the richest hospital in the Durham diocese. It had a gross annual income of £186 0s. 10d., 25% of which was spent on alms. This was about the average for those northern hospitals with a yearly income exceeding £20. Greatham actually devoted 33% to charitable purposes, but Sherburn's contribution of 6% was meagre.

It seems likely that Kepier's income was lessened, as its staff was smaller than that stipulated by Puiset. Choirs were now maintained in some Durham hospitals - Sherburn, Greatham[50] - and at Kepier there were four choral chaplains, William Brymley, Richard and Nicholas Forster and John Gretehede. They were 'continually celebrating and ministering in the said hospital', for which they received a yearly salary of £5 6s 8d. They must have had other duties also - John Gretehede, for instance, is recorded as being steward of the manor of Frosterley in October 1537, when the manor court was held in his presence.[51] There were also two lay clerks, John Blarton and George Scampion, 'daily ministering and singing in the chapel' at an annual payment of £4 each.

None of Puiset's lay-brethren remained. In time, the religious life imposed upon them failed to attract enough capable volunteers. By 1535 it had become customary for monasteries and other religious houses to place the management of their estates in the hands of officials who were of the country gentry class. The chief of these was the high steward, chosen to look after the house's interests at court and elsewhere. The high steward of Kepier was Sir John Bulmer, the head of an important North Yorkshire family.

For his services he received a yearly fee of £3 6s. 8d.[52]

The receivers, who collected the rents, were also country gentry. John Franklyn, a nephew of the master, was the receiver-general at Kepier.[53] Another of his duties was to preside over the manor court of Gilligate. His fee was £4 10s. per annum.

Anthony Wilkinson was the bailiff of St Giles and received a fee of 13s. 4d a year for his supervision of the manor.

All of these gentlemen could claim free board and lodging whenever they needed it, and were therefore a cause of additional expense. Nevertheless, they were almost certainly a benefit to the hospital, as it was in their own interests to make sure that its lands were well-managed.[54]

William Franklyn, the master, had been appointed in 1515. He was chancellor of the diocese, receiver of the bishop's revenues and archdeacon of Durham, besides being rector of Houghton-le-Spring, among other preferments.[55] He must have been away from Kepier often, only staying there when it suited him. Such men, and the patrons who appointed them, contributed to the decline of hospitals all over the country. This led to the closure of many of them and Franklyn was, in fact, the last master of Kepier.

The wayfaring poor were still coming to the hospital gates for the usual distributions of food and drink and, at this stage, even a little money. Some of these were given out daily, some weekly and others on the anniversaries of the founders, all at a cost of £13 a year. In addition to this, further doles to the value of £3 5s. were issued on the anniversaries of benefactors.

Most hospitals were unable to support their original numbers of inmates because of diminished incomes. Greatham, for instance, founded in 1272 for 40 destitute people, cared for only 13 in 1535. At this time there were ten inmates at Kepier, probably also a reduction in number. This may well have been a result of bad harvests in the years 1519-21, together with, in 1520-2, the severest outbreak of the plague in that century. William Franklyn wrote that, of the 4,000 who died in the Palatinate, 3,000 were in Durham city and Darlington.[56] Even with an attempt at a policy of isolation it is unlikely that Kepier itself escaped the infection and its villages must have been affected. Short of food and agricultural labourers, recovery from such catastrophes would have taken a long time. In 1530 the hospital's annual income was £100[57] so that perhaps the improvement made by 1535 was approaching normality.

The practice of paying the inmates in money, instead of providing food and clothing, was generally accepted in 1535. By doing this the negligent or busy master could transfer his responsibilities to the almsmen, who might be too infirm to look after themselves adequately. At Kepier an allowance of £3 a year was paid to each of the ten inmates; this would supply them with necessities, although at a low level of subsistence (the poorest stipendiary curates or chantry priests were working for £4 per annum at this time[58]). Of the many men who received a final home at Kepier these are the only ones whose names are known: William Brantyngham, William Browne, John Chamber (senior and junior), William Crosseby, John Golland, Henry Hawden, Richard Redehede, Christopher Taillior and Martyn Walton. They were clearly old men of the locality as their nine surnames continued to appear in the parish records of succeeding years.

## 19. THE CLOSING OF THE HOSPITAL

After studying the information contained in the Valor Ecclesiasticus Henry VIII ordered the closure of the lesser monastic houses - those with incomes of less than £200 a year. In the north of England this led to the ill-fated uprising known as the Pilgrimage of Grace. Bishop Cuthbert Tunstal, who had acknowledged Henry VIII as Supreme Head of the Church in England, was alarmed and he fled to his castle at Norham, which was held for him by his archdeacon, William Franklyn.[59]

The hospital must have followed the example of its master and offered no support to the Pilgrims. Its steward, Sir John Bulmer, however, together with most of the gentry of the bishopric, joined them. In October 1536 he was one of those who led a force of 5,000 men through Yorkshire to combine with the main host at Pontefract. At the beginning of December the Pilgrims' representatives met the Duke of Norfolk at Doncaster, when they were given the king's pardon and persuaded to disperse. Some arrests were made later and by May 1537 all the principal leaders were prisoners in the Tower. Most of them were condemned to death and Sir John Bulmer was hanged at Tyburn on 25 May for his part in the insurrection. This was ominous news for the community at Kepier. Even so, the master and brethren showed where their sympathies lay by filling the vacant post of steward with another member of the Bulmer family. William Bulmer, presumably Sir John's youngest brother, was recorded as being the steward in 1542.[60]

The failure of the Pilgrimage encouraged Henry VIII to take the greater monasteries into his possession. Towards the end of 1537 or early in 1538 St Cuthbert's shrine was pulled down and its treasures removed. After that no more pilgrims came to Durham. This immediately affected the hospital at Kepier and caused anxiety to both staff and inmates. Their forebodings must have increased when the cathedral priory was dissolved on 31 December 1539, for the priory's own hospitals, Witton Gilbert and St Mary Magdalen, were probably closed at the same time.

The Act of 1539 which legalised the dissolution of the greater monasteries also granted to the Crown those colleges and hospitals which had already been surrendered or which should be surrendered in time to come. The implied threat in this drove many hospitals to give themselves up to the king during the next few years. On 14 January 1544/5 two of the king's agents, Roland Leighton and ' ─────── Rockesbie', rode to Kepier. Received by William Franklyn and 'the fellows' in the hall, the document of surrender would have been formally sealed and handed over. Then the king's men departed under the fearful gaze of the handful of inmates who were left. Later they claimed ten pounds for their costs in going to Kepier.[61]

There was no consistent plan for the future of the hospitals.[62] In county Durham five, including Greatham and Sherburn, were spared, but Kepier was suppressed, along with Staindrop and St Edmund the Bishop at Gateshead. The likeliest reason for the closure of Kepier was the fact that its wealth, as entered in the Valor, was noticed by Sir William Paget, one of the two principal secretaries of state. A man of humble birth, he now saw his chance of becoming a member of the landed gentry by obtaining the Kepier estates for himself. In this purpose he met opposition from Bishop Tunstal, who doubtless had another recipient in view. On 2 February Paget wrote to Sir Ralph Sadler, the other principal secretary, about the matter:

> 'I may tell it you, it has cost me 2,000 marks [£1,333 6s 8d], and forbecause I heard that my lord of Durham was patron and founder of [the hospital] . . . I was desirous to have him made privy to it, and that the thing might pass with his consent. . . . He hath answered nay . . . The denial of it shall not hinder the proceedings thereof, but only be a signification to the King's Majesty how my said lord misliketh his Highness' doings in those things.[63]'

Paget was one of the king's most trusted advisers and he was able to use his influence to secure the desired property for himself. On 6 February he was granted 'the hospital of St Giles of Kepier beside Durham and all its possessions' in Durham, Northumberland and Yorkshire. The new proprietor also had the advowson of those churches which had been appropriated to the hospital - St Giles' and St Nicholas' in Durham, and St James', Hunstanworth. In future, the incumbents of these churches would be appointed by Paget and further lay successors. For his elevation to the ranks of landowners Paget paid £1,000 into the king's own hands and £333 6s 8d to the Court of Augmentations, which dealt with the property of the dissolved houses. Besides this down payment there was also an annual rent of £16 15s. 1d.[64]

In the document recording the purchase of Kepier the name of Richard Cox, professor of theology, was associated with that of Paget. It seems that Dr Cox was simply a supporter of Paget in his request, because he paid no money for the property and is not heard of again in connection with it. He was at that time tutor to Prince Edward and godfather to Paget's eldest son.[65]

Paget was a close friend of the Earl of Hertford (later Protector Somerset), who was in the north preparing for a military campaign in Scotland during the summer of 1545. A 'scarcity of victuals and other things at Newcastle' forced him to return to Darlington in the hope of raising better supplies there. On arrival he wrote to Paget:

> '... I took horse hitherwards yesterday; and, between Newcastle and Durham, received your letter to me and another to your chaplain at Kepier, whereupon I went to your house there, delivered your letter and took upon me the part of a surveyor. It is not to be greatly esteemed, but the situation and commodities are such as I wish were near London. ... Darlington, 14 June 1545.'[66]

The letter makes it clear that Paget had not seen Kepier (having been in the Low Countries from February to late April, before returning to London) and that one of the chaplains had been retained to act in some supervisory or secretarial capacity.

It is reasonable to suppose that Richard Forster was the chaplain alluded to and that he continued to live at Kepier for many more years. According to his will, written on 6 September 1575, his master was Anthony Middleton, a witness of the will. This gentleman had had an early connection with the dissolved hospital and was steward of the manor of Gilesgate by at least 1555. In that year he was referred to as 'of Kepier', so it would seem that he and his family had their home in part of the old hospital buildings. He bought the estate of Newton Hall in 1565, but was still steward of the Gilesgate manor in 1579. He died in 1581 and was buried in St Margaret's church. Richard Forster died soon after making his will, desiring to be buried on 'the left hand of my father whereas he lyeth' in a church the name of which can no longer be read. However, the parish register of St Nicholas' church states that 'Richard Forster, Priest', was 'buried within the church doors' on 14 September. He left a considerable amount of money and goods, his bequests including shillings for the poor of the parishes of St Giles, St Margaret and Elvet (possibly St Nicholas, too - the words are obliterated), as well as for the prisoners in Durham, 'to get them meat'. There were also keepsakes for Anthony Middleton, his son and daughter and small token sums of money to other members of the family. Richard Forster presents an interesting link between the hospital and its subsequent history under lay ownership.[67]

Paget almost certainly never visited his northern possession. Remembering Hertford's comment about its distance from London, he found a more desirable property nearer the capital. On 23 January 1545/6 he sold the hospital estates to the Crown. In exchange for this, 'and for his services', the king granted him the house and site of the late college of Burton upon Trent, Staffordshire, with its manors and other lands, on 31 January 1545/6. He had thus held Kepier for less than a year before it reverted to Henry VIII.[68]

The manor court would then have been held in the name of the king and a royal steward appointed to look after his interests. Edward VI, succeeding his father in January 1546/7, leased the Kepier estates for a term of 21 years from 4 August 1547[69] to John Franklyn, once the receiver-general of the hospital.

Indications of the lives of three other former hospital staff-members can be seen in certain records: John Gretehede, prebendary of Eldon (College of Auckland) in 1535, was receiving a pension for this post in 1553,[70] Nicholas Forster was a chaplain of Henry, Earl of Westmorland, and parson of Brancepeth in 1563, when the earl made his will leaving him £20 - he probably remained at Brancepeth till 1571, when George Cliffe became the rector;[71] John Blarton, with 'my godmother his wife', was left 6s 8d and one load of wheat in the will of John Franklyn, then of Cocken, and he also witnessed the will, November 1572. He had become the parish clerk of Houghton-le-Spring and, according to his will, made in May 1582, wished to be buried in 'our parish churchyard of Houghton'. Dying soon afterwards he left 'portions' to his four children and the term of the lease of his house equally between two of them.[72] No trace has been found of William Brimley or George Scampion.

The master, William Franklyn, had other preferments for his support. Since December 1536 he had been Dean of Windsor (in which appointment he had assisted at the christening of Edward VI in October 1537). In 1552 he retired to his rectory of Chalfont St Giles, Buckinghamshire, where he died in January 1555/56 and was buried in the church there.[73]

One clause in the Act for the Dissolution of the Lesser Monasteries (1536) stated that those who came into possession of the lands of religious houses should supply hospitality and service for the poor, as was formerly done.[74] This seemed a natural provision, especially in the case of the hospitals, whose founders and benefactors had made their gifts specifically for the purpose of supporting the poor and sick. The new owners of hospital buildings, however, do not appear to have considered the fate of the inmates to have been their responsibility. Sir William Paget would have had no need to provide for the few remaining inmates at Kepier, forlorn victims of a grasping king's covetousness. It is not known what happened to them - perhaps they were transferred to the unsuppressed hospital at Sherburn. In this way the charitable work of Kepier came to an end.

For four centuries the hospital had been a final home to many of the local poor and infirm and a temporary resting-place for generations of pilgrims and wayfarers. After 1545 it remained only as a faint memory in old men's minds, symbol of a seemingly golden time gone forever, a building which now welcomed the new rich and to whose gates travellers no longer bent their weary footsteps at the setting of the sun.

## 20. LAY OWNERS

It must have taken some time for the people of Durham and the tenants of the hospital to accustom themselves to the change in use and ownership of Kepier. As late as 1613 Thomas Wall, recently deceased, was said to have held the Wester Peackefeild at Frosterley 'of the hospital of Kepier'.[75] It was then 68 years since the closure and subsequently there had been three lay owners.

**John Cockburn**

Edward VI granted the hospital to John Cockburn, Lord of Ormiston, subject to the lease made to John Franklyn in 1547. This gentleman was one of many Scotsmen who were in favour of an alliance with England through a marriage between the boy king, Edward VI, and the child Mary, Queen of Scots. With others, he served the English cause faithfully, often at great danger to himself, his retainers and possessions - in February 1548 his house at Ormiston in East Lothian had been destroyed and the occupants of it executed.

On 12 May 1552 Cockburn and his wife, Alison, together with their children, Alexander, John, Barbara and Sibyl, were granted English citizenship. Furthermore, on 23 May, he was rewarded by 'the gift . . . of the Hospital of Kepier . . . with all the lands, profits and commodities to the same belonging . . . in consideration of his good service and losses sustained by [him].' The estate provided Cockburn with an income but, because of John Franklyn's lease, he was not able to live at Kepier. His wife and children were with him for, on 14 October 1551, a letter was sent from the Privy Council to the Mayor of Newcastle and others, requiring them 'to see the Lord Ormiston furnished of a meet lodging to lay his wife in at the time of her delivery of child. . . .' The lodging provided would appear to have been the house of the Greyfriars at Newcastle because, on 11 December 1552, Cockburn was asked to give the house up to its owner, Sir Marmaduke Tunstall. The unsettled life he led made it difficult for him to have a permanent abode. Nevertheless he was lord of the manor of Gilligate and at some time between 12 May 1552 and 25 March 1554/5 he agreed to the moving of 'a beautiful marble cross' from the upper part of Gilesgate to the market place in Durham.

At the beginning of 1555 Cockburn, who was a devoted supporter of the reformed faith, was in some sort of trouble with the government of the Catholic Mary I and he tried to escape to Scotland. Arrested on the Border, he was imprisoned in Norham castle. The Bishop of Durham was directed to keep him in custody until he had repaid £500 said to be owing to the Crown; also to find out 'what he hath done with the rest of the money which he received for the hospital by him sold.' Cockburn had, in fact, found a buyer in a London merchant called John Heath. It is possible that these two men had met on one of the Scotsman's visits to his political masters in London; and that Cockburn had invited John Heath to look at his Kepier possessions with a view to buying them. In the attempt to leave England in a hurry he must have been ready to make a quick sale so that, on 25 March, John Heath was able to buy at a bargain price.

In September Cockburn was sent up to London and kept in the Fleet prison until December, when he was called before the Privy Council. No evidence was brought against him, 'and so was discharged of further imprisonment.' He returned to Scotland although his association with the English continued in the reign of Elizabeth I.[76]

Seeing that the hospital was temporarily vacant the lord treasurer commanded Richard Ashton, the receiver there, to remove and sell 'certain lead upon thospitall of Kepyer'. This lead would have been from the roof of the chapel and infirmary. It had been given by

Puiset nearly 400 years before, although doubtless patched up from time to time since then. The next owner was to find part of his buildings only recently robbed for the benefit of the royal coffers.[77]

**The Heath Family**

On 20 June 1555 the manor court of Gilesgate was held in the name of John Heath, the new occupier of Kepier. He had surely bought the property as an investment and looked to climb higher in the social scale. In the manor court held on 17 January 1557/8 he was referred to as John Heath 'armiger' (i.e. one entitled to a coat of arms), although the grant of arms was not confirmed till 4 August. He and his son, John, would have ridden north from time to time to collect revenues and to survey the former hospital territories. They were so impressed that the son decided to settle at Kepier when John Franklyn's lease expired in August 1568.[78]

The younger John Heath was a successful merchant and a member of the London coopers' company. On 6 June 1558 he had bought the wardenship of the Fleet prison, a superior position of trust with many opportunities, through fees and rents, of financial gain. In January of the following year he sold the wardenship, assuredly at a profit. By 1563 he had removed to Norfolk, where he was described as 'of London, now of King's Lynn'. The next few years saw steady preparations for the migration to Durham so that he was ready to enter Kepier shortly after John Franklyn had departed. With him he brought his second wife, Thomasine, his eldest son, John, with his wife Elizabeth and their first child, another John (b. 1568), son Nicholas and Edward, at least one daughter and his unmarried sister, Agnes. There was plenty of room in the old hospital buildings for all of them and Kepier was soon looked on as their home.

The Rising of the North occurred in November 1569 when former Catholic ways of worship were revived briefly in Durham. This must have troubled John Heath who was a supporter of the reformed religion and whose father was patron of both St Giles' and St Nicholas' churches. However, the rebellion was suppressed by Christmas and nothing else disturbed the southern family on the banks of the Wear. Its members were quickly accepted into the society of their northern neighbours and, in time, one daughter married a well-to-do city merchant, Henry Smith, and two grandsons married daughters of the country gentry. John Heath himself came to be on friendly terms with senior diocesan clergy.[79]

John Heath of London had died by 11 September 1573 and the son who was already living in Durham succeeded to the Kepier estates.[80] Since coming to Durham 'John Heath of Kepier' had met Bernard Gilpin, rector of Houghton-le-Spring, and the two shared a desire to advance the Protestant faith in the north. They discussed the founding of a 'godly grammar school' for the training of able teachers for the Church, and also an almshouse, both to be near Gilpin's church. Heath offered to provide generous endowments for this endeavour out of the Kepier lands. In an agreement dated 24 September 1570 he began by conveying to the Dean and Chapter pensions from certain rectories as well as gillytithes in Bishop Wearmouth, Cleadon, Easington and Chester-le-Street, to be used for the payment of a schoolmaster and an usher. Should Bernard Gilpin obtain the Queen's charter of incorporation for the school and the almshouse these would be passed to the corporation.

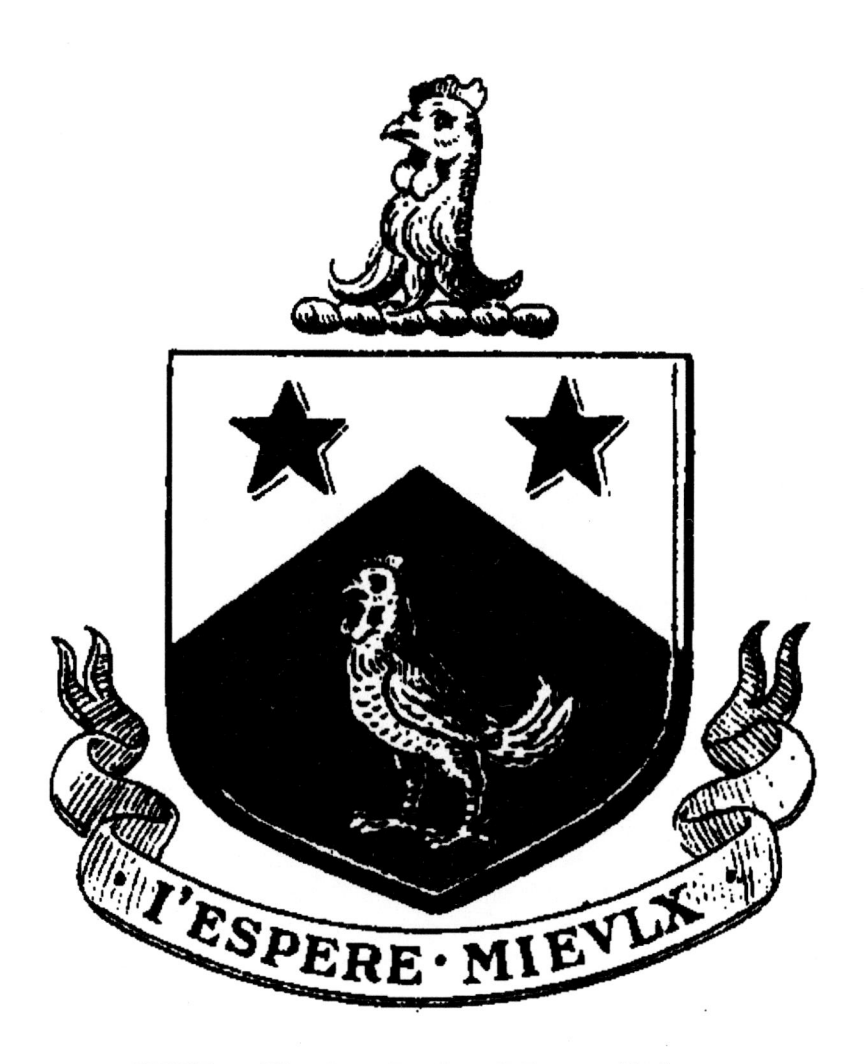

## HEATH OF KEPIER.

*ARMS: Party per chev. or and sa., in chief two mullets, in base a heath-cock wattled gu., countercharged.*

*CREST: On a wreath, a heath-cock's head erased sa., wattled gu.*

16. Heath of Kepier. Arms: party per chevron or and sable, in chief 2 mullets, in base a heath-cock wattled gules, counterchanged. Crest: on a wreath, a heath-cocks head erased sable, wattled gules.

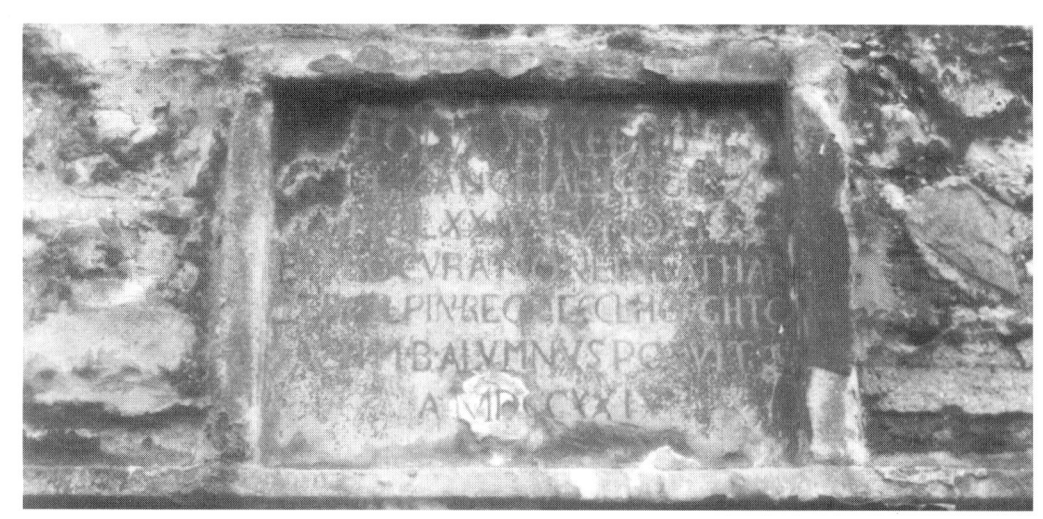

*M. F. Richardson*

17. Houghton-le-Spring old grammer school: inscription by Christopher Hunter, dated 1724, commemorating the founding of the school by John Heath and Bernard Gilpin in 1574.

Letters patent were sealed on 2 April 1574. Both school and almshouse were named 'Kepier', from the source of the endowments and to honour the benefactor. Gilpin and Heath were named as the first two governors with power to appoint others. This right was vested in the subsequent rectors of Houghton and heirs of Heath. (On the eighteenth-century school-house a stone records the munificence of John Tempest, who was a later governor and a descendant of John Heath.) The lay founder's interest was maintained and, by his will, dated 28 August 1589, he left £40 'to the maintenance of the poorest or aptest scholars who shall go to Oxford or Cambridge from Kepier School'.

After a long and distinguished history the school closed in 1922. The original building remains, although put to other uses. Over the doorway is a Latin inscription commemorating the foundation. On it the names of B. Gilpin and J. Heath can still be read. The almshouse was not built until after the time of the founders.[81]

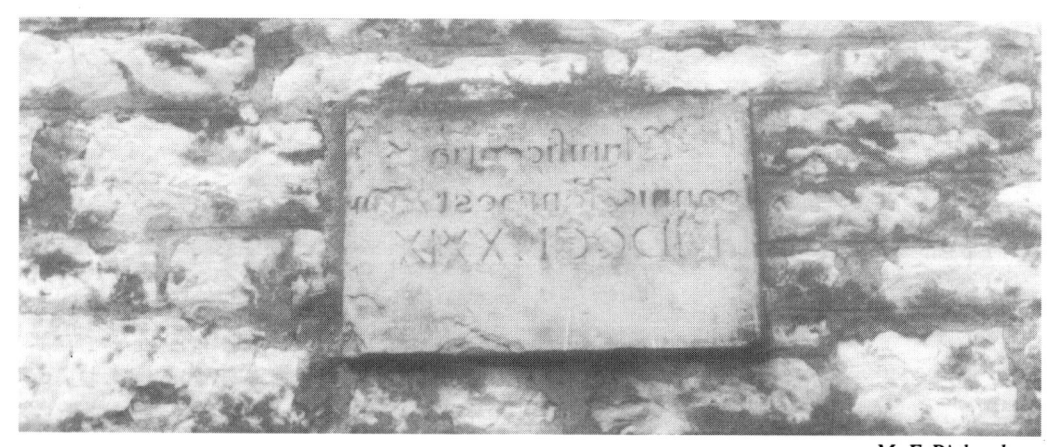

*M. F. Richardson,*

18. Houghton-le-Spring old grammar school: John Tempest commemorative inscription, 1779.

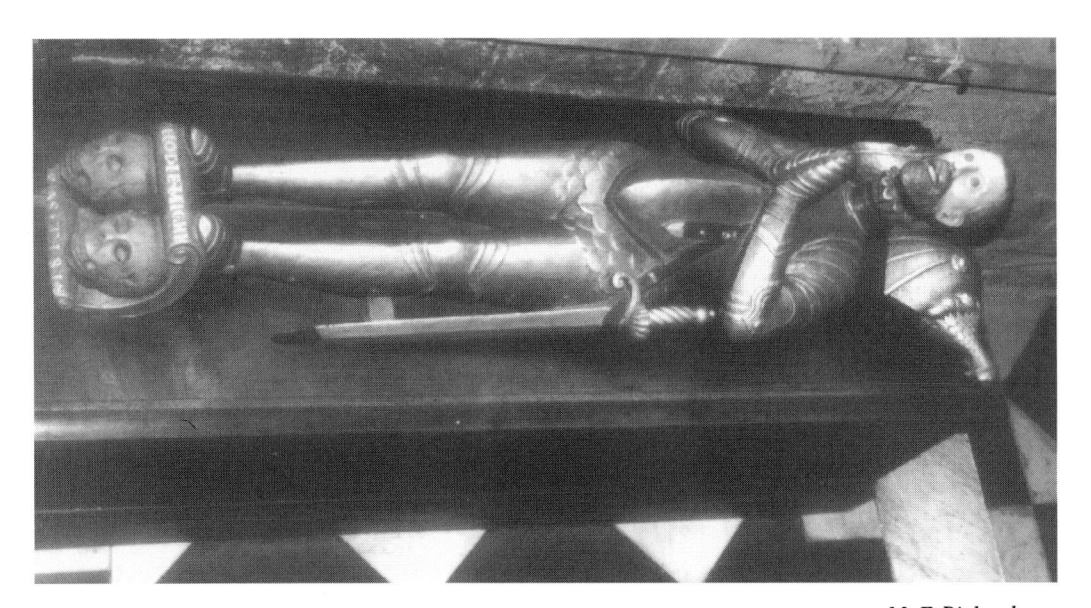

M. F. Richardson
19. St Giles church: recumbent effigy of John Heath (d. 1590), wearing plate armour and with the head on a tilting helmet surmounted by his cock's head crest.

John Heath was patron of St Giles' church and many family baptisms, marriages and burials took place there. He himself was buried in the chancel on 11 August 1590. His wooden recumbent effigy in Elizabethan armour lies on a tomb-chest of later date. He had parted with several of the distant properties of the hospital, but kept intact the lands at Kepier and Old Durham. In his will he made the first division of the Kepier property by leaving Ramside grange (on the eastern edge of the estate, here mentioned for the first time) to his youngest son, Edward.[82]

The eldest son, John, is thought to have been the builder of a grand, modern house for his family. To make room for it he cleared the south side of the courtyard where the roofless chapel and infirmary may once have stood, remaining only as a ruin. Then a fine mansion of brick, with a stone loggia on the ground floor of the south front, was raised (the stone being almost certainly re-used from the hospital site). The fashionable loggia may be compared with the one built in Durham market place in 1617 round the marble cross (see page xx above); and also the arcade of similar date added to the front of the medieval Bradley Hall, near Wolsingham. 'The warm red of the thin bricks, contrasted with the browns and yellows of the stonework, must have given a fine effect.'

The interior was described by Boyle in 1892 as having a 'broad, balustered oak staircase' leading up to the great hall, the walls of which were 'covered with the remains of once splendidly carved panelling'. Forty years later those who had seen it remembered that 'no two panels were alike.' A lawn and gardens were laid out to the south of the house, with a small orchard on the eastern slope and pear trees espaliered against the west-facing wall of an enclosure on the west side of the house near the road. The entire setting was surrounded by a high brick wall. To sit within the stone arcade on a summer evening and

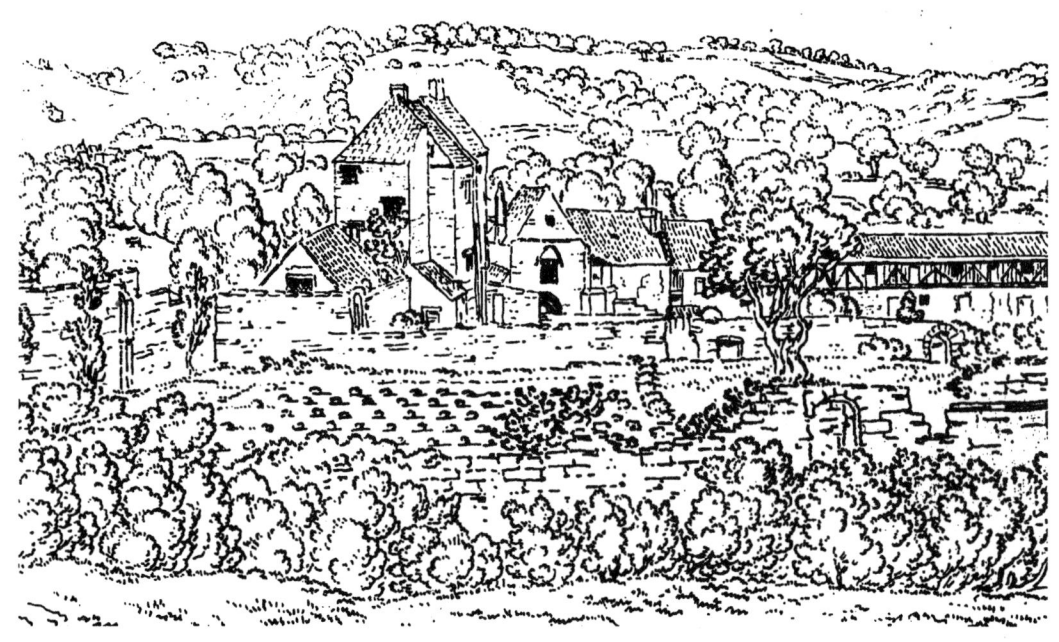

*S. H. Grimm*

20. Kepier: Panorama view from the east.

admire the view, to saunter between the flower-beds and to pluck the fruit in autumn would have afforded a new-found pleasure to the occupants and their guests. Here was a residence of which a gentleman might be proud.[83]

John Heath, the second of that name to live at Kepier, was disappointed in the thriftless behaviour of his eldest son and heir, another John, and apparently gave the West and East Granges to the more reliable second son, Thomas. By his will, made 24 November 1612, he put limitations on what John might do with the Kepier estate. John owed his father the large sum of £500 and the bills proving this were left to Thomas. Payment would only be demanded if John should make 'waste of the woods belonging to the premises' or dig 'any mines for coals' or fail to 'repair and keep up all the houses in his possession.'[84] This was the state of affairs when the second John Heath died in January 1617/8.

John Heath the third's only child, a boy called Thomas, had died in 1594 and his brother was therefore his heir. Thomas does not seem to have had a sentimental attachment to the family home at Kepier, but was content with living at the East Grange. An agreement was made between the two brothers by which John relinquished his rights in the Durham estate and Thomas became the lord of the manor of Gilesgate. The first entry in the Manor Court Book, beginning October 1634, records that the court is held in the name of Thomas Heath. Similar entries continue up to 1654.[85]

On 29 December 1629 Thomas and his son John sold the Kepier site. The buyer was Ralph Cole, merchant of Newcastle (who, six years later, also bought Brancepeth castle). He gained the 'mansion-house, gardens, orchard, curtilage, and grange-house [i.e. the West Grange], Kepier mills, Ayreson's farm,' and garths, meadows, orchards, a paddock and a close, besides.[86]

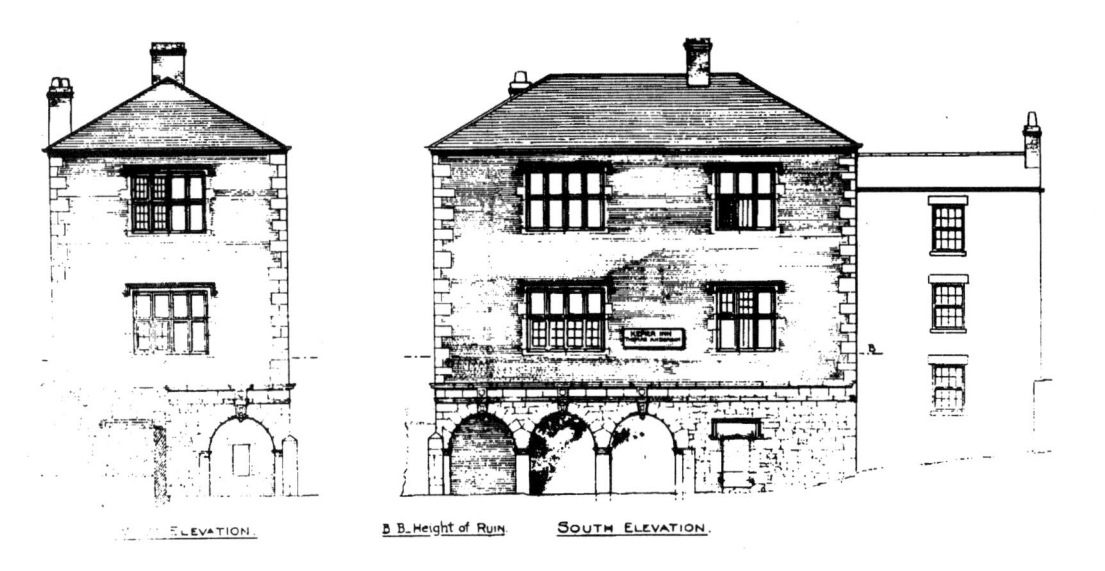

*W. G. Footitt*

21. Heath mansion, 1883-8, then an inn, when Thomas Anderson was inn-keeper. Note surviving leaded panes and Elizabethan loggia still in good condition.

On 18 January 1629/30 a settlement of property was made on Thomas Heath for life and, after his death, on his son John, then of Gray's Inn; and providing for his wife Dorothy to continue to live at the East Grange with an income from the estate. This included the manor of Old Durham. John the elder was still in possession of Old Durham and in February 1630/1 he made a settlement of it on himself for life and the farmstead continued to give him an income.[87]

The last Heath of Kepier spent his remaining years living in the gatehouse, to which his father had added a broad flight of steps and imposing doorway leading to the upper storey. He was not alone for he married again sometime after the death of his first wife in 1631. The furniture and furnishings probably belonged to the time of his grandfather, if not before that, for the inventory taken at his death was long and seems to record the accumulated possessions of decades, many items being described as 'old'. He lived in a certain ancient splendour - there were four carpets on the floor of 'the outer chamber', a canopy bedstead, a press with drawers, a great wainscot chair, four embroidered cushions, a clock, a pair of playing tables, a seeing- glass (i.e. a mirror) and much besides. In 'the chamber over the entry' was a truckle bed with a featherbed, a little table with drawers, a livery cupboard and two desks. 'Topp's chamber' (and Topp Heath - John's cousin - had died in 1620) had a trunk, a Flanders chest and a screen, as well as a bedstead. The study housed John's books on shelves and there was a lantern to assist with reading. There were plenty of tables, chairs, stools, chests, cupboards, curtains and pewter goods and more than enough of household linen and some silver - 'a great Salt and a little Salt', for example; and in 'the brushing chamber' were wool and yarn.

In 'the brewhouse and other houses thereabouts' were a sow and a pig, tools and implements, tubs and barrels, a saddle, bridle and saddle-cloth, a coach and farm cart, hay in the stable and stores of rye and coal.[88]

John Heath made his will on 21 July 1637 and the next year he presented a silver communion cup, with paten, to the church of St Giles. Round the base of the cup is the touching inscription, 'Remember John Hethe esqr the third and last of keepeyre: 1638', and on the paten is the date, 'Desember the: 25th: 1638'. He died on 6 January 1639/40, aged 71, and was buried the next day 'about the fourth hour of the morning'. The reason for this speedy interment is not given but the St Giles' parish register refers to him as 'a pious man, father of the poor and of this church a benefactor'.[89]

Thomas now succeeded to his brother's possessions which included Old Durham. The original lease of this manor to Richard Booth had expired in 1578, but it seems to have been renewed for, when Robert Booth died in 1592, he was still 'of Old Durham'. The 'farmhold' appears to have been leased by the Heaths well into the next century. In 1642 Thomas Heath's son, John (the eventual occupier), was known as 'of the city of Durham', but in 1648 he was recorded as 'of Old Durham.' Between those two dates he had made his home in the old manor house, which he inherited on the death of his father (1654). These facts suggest that he was unable to live at Old Durham at first because it was leased to someone else.[90]

It was probably this John Heath who planned the gardens at Old Durham in emulation of those at Kepier. His initials were seen by Surtees on the summerhouse (or gazebo). Elizabeth, John's only child and heiress, married John Tempest in 1642, when a settlement of the Heath estates was made. When 'John Heath, Esquire, of Old Durham,' died on Sunday 1 March 1664/5 the event and the weather were noted in the letter of a family friend. Because of 'the most violent storm of snow and frost' ever since Christmas there had been 'no stirring from town to town'. These conditions made it difficult for the funeral procession to climb the hill from Old Durham to St Giles' church. The writer continued, 'and at this very day the frost is great, the weather cold, and a great snow. This day we are going to bury Mr. Heath.' John Heath would have been buried in the chancel of the church, as were his predecessors.[91]

Old Durham remained the Tempest family home until the mid-eighteenth century when a move was made to Sherburn Hall and subsequently to Wynyard. Elizabeth Heath's descendant, Frances Anne Vane-Tempest-Stewart, Marchioness of Londonderry, was proud to describe herself as 'Heiress of Heath' on a silver flagon which she presented to the church of St Giles in 1845.[92]

### The Cole Family

During the last ten years of the third John Heath's life Ralph Cole's son, Nicholas, had settled at Kepier and there are references to the family in the baptismal and burial registers of St Giles' church from 1636. Within a few years the pleasures of life at Kepier were interrupted by the outbreak of the Civil War. Nicholas Cole, like most of the upper classes in county Durham (including John Heath and John Tempest) took the Royalist side. Elected mayor of Newcastle in 1640, he was knighted in the same year by Charles I and created a baronet in 1641. Parliament, however, labelled him a 'delinquent', i.e. an adherent of the king. In the defence of Newcastle and the subsequent storming of the town by the Scots in 1644 he, his father and brother were taken prisoner, but Nicholas managed to escape. He was exempted from pardon and did not make his peace with Parliament until 1649. The Coles were heavily fined for their delinquency, Nicholas' fine being completely paid on 20 May 1652 and that of his father on 17 August 1653.[93]

The county of Durham suffered from the presence of both the Scottish and Royalist armies and the 'tenants of Mr. Ralph Cole at Kepier and the Grange' endured losses along with everybody else. In 1644 Thomas Snawdon's meadow grounds were 'all destroyed' by the Scottish troopers; two closes that he farmed were 'eaten with the troopers and 15 acres of oats destroyed.' 150 horses were put into Timothy Hubbuck's 'pasture called Lime Kiln' for two days and nights; the meadow and pasture of Edward Robinson 'of Kepier' were 'all destroyed', although he was able to keep four cows all the summer there; and Mrs Margaret Blakiston, widow, farmed one close of meadow called Craw Orchard, which was 'all destroyed'.[94]

After raising the cash for the payment of their fines neither Sir Nicholas nor Sir Ralph would have had much money left for land improvement. Sir Nicholas died at Kepier in 1669 and was buried at St Giles' on 17 December. Bishop John Cosin, then in London, receiving the news from his secretary, Miles Stapylton. He wrote back on 21 December, 'I am very sorry to hear of Sir Nicholas Cole's sudden death, whereby I have lost a very honest gentleman and a very good neighbour'; he asked Miles Stapylton to go to 'my good Lady Cole' with his condolences. Little more than four years later Cole's younger son, another Nicholas, also died at Kepier.[95]

The decayed condition of the property may have been a contributory factor to leading his elder brother, Sir Ralph of Brancepeth, to sell the Kepier estate to Sir Christopher Musgrave of Carlisle in 1674.[96]

**The Musgrave family**
The Musgraves seem to have treated Kepier as an investment. They never lived there but supervised from afar through a land agent. The mansion house, gatehouse and mill would have been let to tenants.[97]

**Kepier Gardens**
The gardens created by the second John Heath continued to be carefully tended and were now an amenity for the neighbourhood. When that adventurous lady, Celia Fiennes, who was touring England on horseback, came to Durham in July or August 1698, she also visited Kepier:

> '... in walking by this river [the Wear] we came to Sir Charles Musgrave's house which is now old and ruinous but has been good; the gardens are flourishing still with good walks and much fruit of which I tasted. It's a place that is used like our Spring Gardens for the Company of the town to walk in the evening and it's most pleasant by the river....'[98]

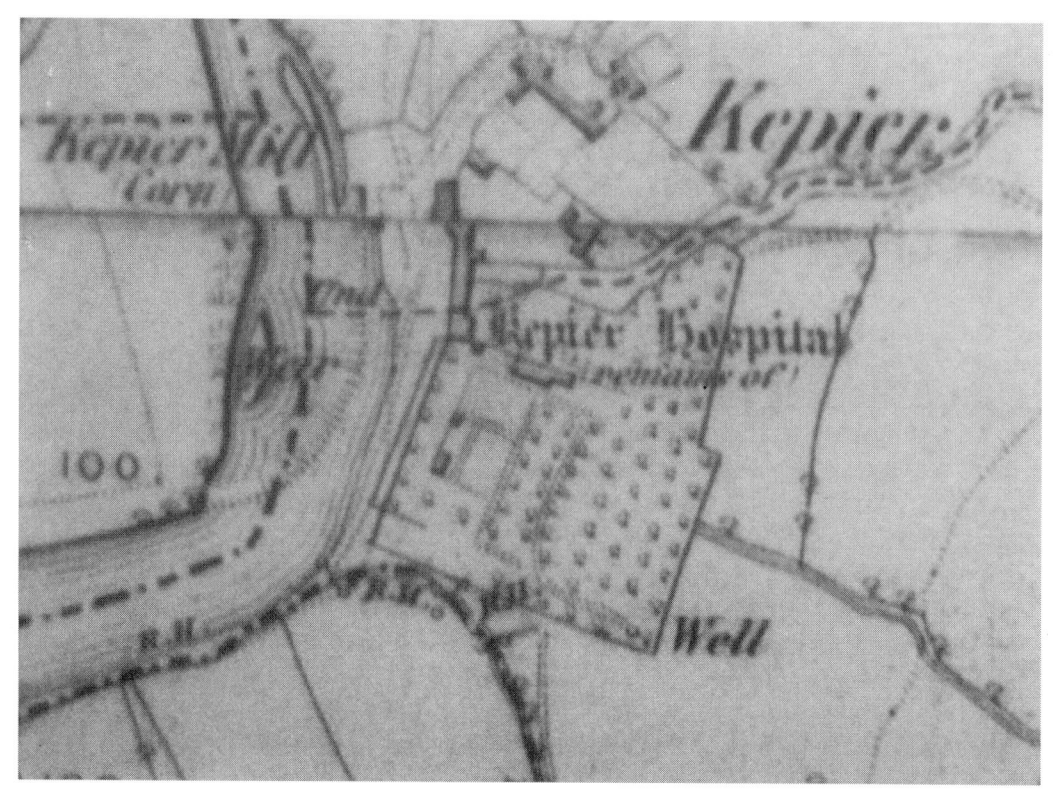

*M. F. Richardson*
22. Kepier garden plan from the Ordinance Survey of 1858. Note the site of two summer houses and the pear orchard on the east side sloping towards the garden plots.

    The gardens seem to have been let to proprietors, like William Robinson of Kepier. Although called a gardener in his will, made in December 1752, he was a wealthy man, owning burgages and separate plots of land in Gilesgate. He would have employed men to do the work of the soil. The public, presumably, was charged for admission to the gardens. In the early part of the eighteenth century 'the tradesmen of the town were wont to resort thither at sundry times during the summer months to regale themselves'. Sometimes a part of the riverside road from Durham might crumble into the river, creating danger for unwary foot-passengers. On one occasion Thomas Brockett, a respectable plumber, narrowly escaped drowning after returning from spending an afternoon 'amid the shaded walks of Kepier'.[99]

### Two artists at Kepier
    The decaying beauty of the old hospital attracted two notable artists in the late eighteenth century within a few years of each other. Samuel Hieronymous Grimm, who was living in Durham between 1777 and 1784, drew three sketches of Kepier - the gatehouse, both from the outside and from the courtyard, and a panoramic view from the east includ-

ing the Heath mansion and the building which is now the present farmhouse. The timber-framed row with its pantiles is evident, as well as garden walls becoming ruinous, a view of the north and east sides with a small garden plot, and over all an air of romantic neglect.

William Beilby, 'the greatest glass decorator of all time', was born in Durham in 1740 and would have known Kepier. He left for Gateshead and eventual fame as a glass-painter at the age of 19. During a brief return made some time between 1774 and 1778, when he was already well-known, he painted a charming water-colour of the west side of the gate-house. An additional reason for his interest in the old place may have been a slight family connection. Mary Heath, a descendant of the first John Heath of Kepier by his fourth son, Nicholas, married a James Beilby of Scarborough, afterwards of South Shields, in 1759. The water-colour is unique in showing the close on the right of the gateway with the pear trees trained against the wall and an entrance to it, with steps down, from the main grounds of the house.

The Musgraves must have let the farm land at Kepier to a tenant-farmer. Rob Rutherford was called 'Late farmer at Kepier' on his headstone which can be seen in Pittington churchyard. He died in October 1804 aged 73. The names of his three sons, Stephen, Rob and James, who had all died before him, are inscribed on the same stone. It is possible that he was at Kepier when the two artists visited it. In one of Grimm's drawings the old courtyard looks very like a farmyard with its large hayrick and half a dozen ducks. The figure sitting by a door north of the gatehouse may well be one of Rob Rutherford's sons.[100]

## Kepier Inn

By 1827 the mansion house had become an inn called the 'White Bear' or 'Kepier Inn'. It was visited in 1841 by three young brothers, descendants of Nicholas Heath and great-nephews of Mary Heath, mentioned above. They were making a tour of ancestral properties and the eldest of them, John Carlen Heath, wrote in his account of their outing:

'. . . it is somewhat fortunate for preserving the traditions connected with the places, that Kepier and Old Durham are now popular summer resorts, for the hosts and the customers naturally get on to discourse of the former conditions of the houses and to whom they belonged.'

With their surname they probably received an extra special welcome.[101]

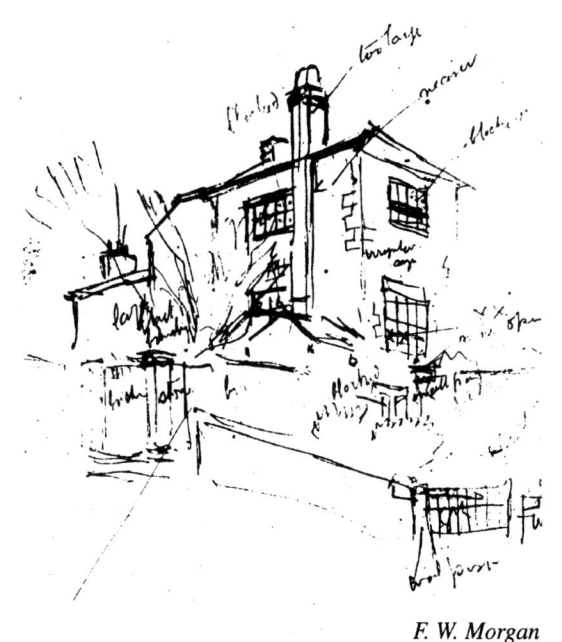

*F. W. Morgan*
23. Heath mansion from the north-west, c. 1887, demolished 1892. *(By courtesy of The British Architectural Library, RIBA, London).*

*M. F. Richardson*

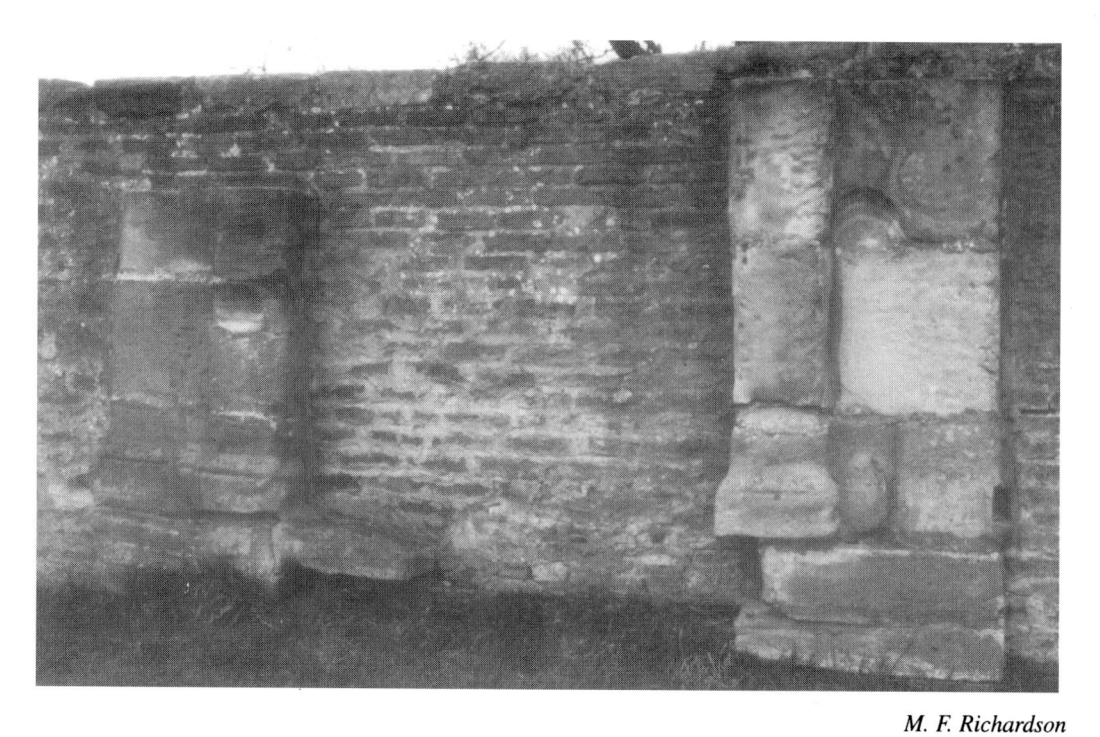

24. Bricked up gateway to the Heath mansion grounds.

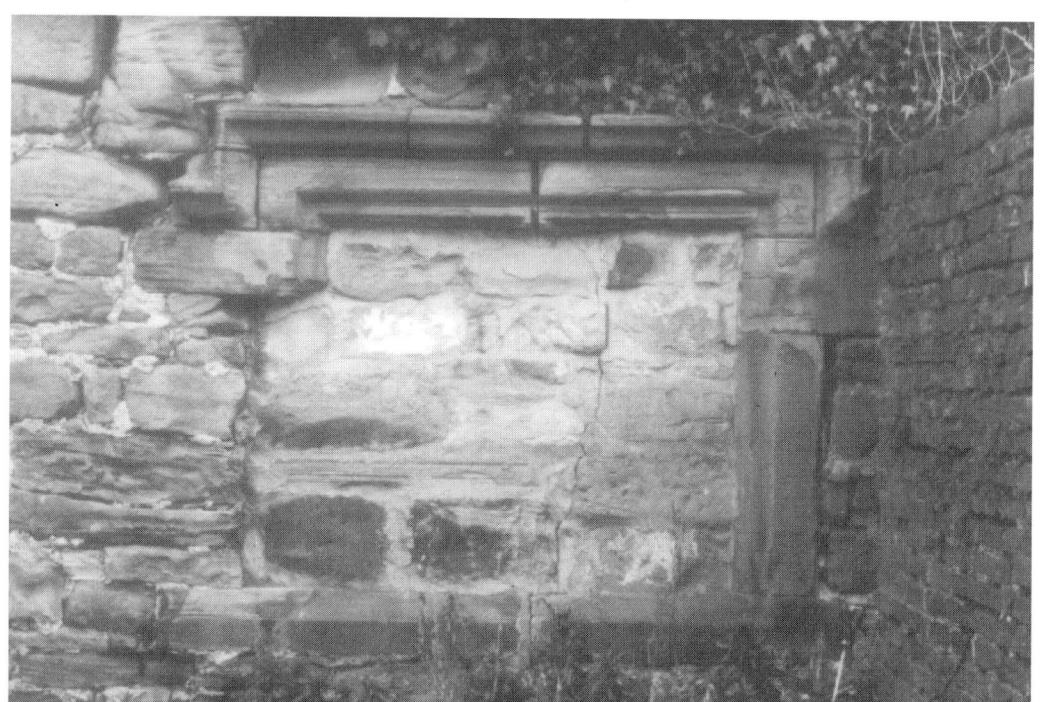

*M. F. Richardson*

25. Blocked window in the west wall of the Kepier mansion.

## Kepier Mill

It is likely that the ancient duty of individuals to grind their corn in the manorial mill at Kepier had ceased to be enforced in the 1600s. Parallels for this can be found in other places.[102] Even so, in 1640 the Cole family instituted a suit in the Durham Court of Chancery to establish the facts of the matter. Somehow the defendants managed to prove that no such custom had existed (meaning, perhaps, since the closure of the hospital). From that time it was clear that they could not be compelled to use the mill.[103]

The hard work of being a miller was recompensed by a satisfactory income. John Banks, miller of Kepier, who made his will in December 1700, bequeathed three houses in Gilesgate to his wife Anne, as well as a close 'commonly called Porter Close'. When he died two years later he was buried in the nave of St Giles' church. His memorial slab was noticed in 1834, although it has since been removed.[104]

The job had its dangers and at least two millers died going about their business. In 1705 'John Coulson, mill-wright and miller of Kepier corn mills [died] suddenly by a fall on the causeway over against his own house early in the morning (being on foot and leading a horse to water)'; and John Airson, possibly his successor, 'was drowned in his dam', in July 1713.[105]

A flourishing business kept the mill-wheels turning and the roads to Kepier would have been busy with carters going to and fro with their corn and flour. When the great house became an inn it must have benefited from this passing trade.

All came to an end, however, on Saturday 24 September 1870, when the mill was totally destroyed by fire. The Durham Chronicle gave a vivid account of what happened:[106]

> 'The mill, it appeared, had been working overnight. Young Stonehouse [son of the miller, George Stonehouse] was left to work the mill, while his father was sleeping in one of the apartments of the building. Young Stonehouse had fallen asleep at his task. On awakening at a quarter to three, after a very short slumber, he found the building filled with smoke. At once apprehending the cause, he went out to procure pails of water, and, on returning, he was overcome by the smoke, and fell down from its effects. He, however, managed to make his escape, and with some difficulty, succeeded in arousing his father . . . Mr. Stonehouse was naturally very much alarmed, but he succeeded, not without great difficulty, in getting out of the mill, the fire having by this time made considerable headway. It was not until four o'clock that the borough engine . . . arrived on the spot. It was then impossible to save the mill or any portion of it; but with a view to the protection of property in the immediate vicinity, the engine commenced to play on the burning mass, and this operation was continued for some hours . . . The roof fell in about four o'clock, and soon nothing but the bare walls remained of the mill. At seven o'clock, one of those walls gave way and fell, several persons standing about having a narrow escape. It is stated that the fire was caused by 'overworking the mill, through pressure of business'. In order to produce meal of the required description, it was necessary to have the stones placed

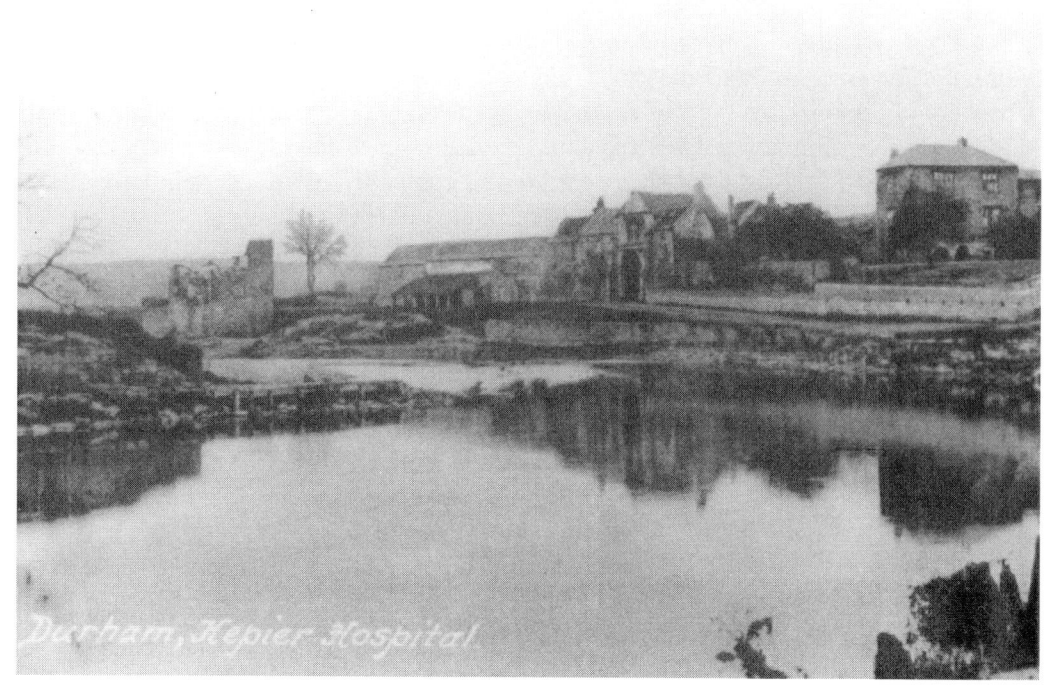

26. Kepier: general view.  
Late 19th-century postcard

very close to each other, and the grinding together of the stones caused sparks to be thrown off, which in course of time, set on fire the wood-work surrounding the wheels. There was plenty of wood and other material to feed the flames, which soon spread with rapidity, resulting in the complete destruction of the building. Neither the property nor the stock (which, it is said, included one hundred sacks of meal), were covered by insurance. Mr. Walton, agent for Sir George Musgrave, visited Kepier in the course of the morning. On Sunday last, some hundreds of residents of this city had a stroll to Kepier for the purpose of inspecting the ruins.'

The mill was never rebuilt. The roofless, empty shell gradually disintegrated through the following years. Only the arch above the mill-stream can be seen today.

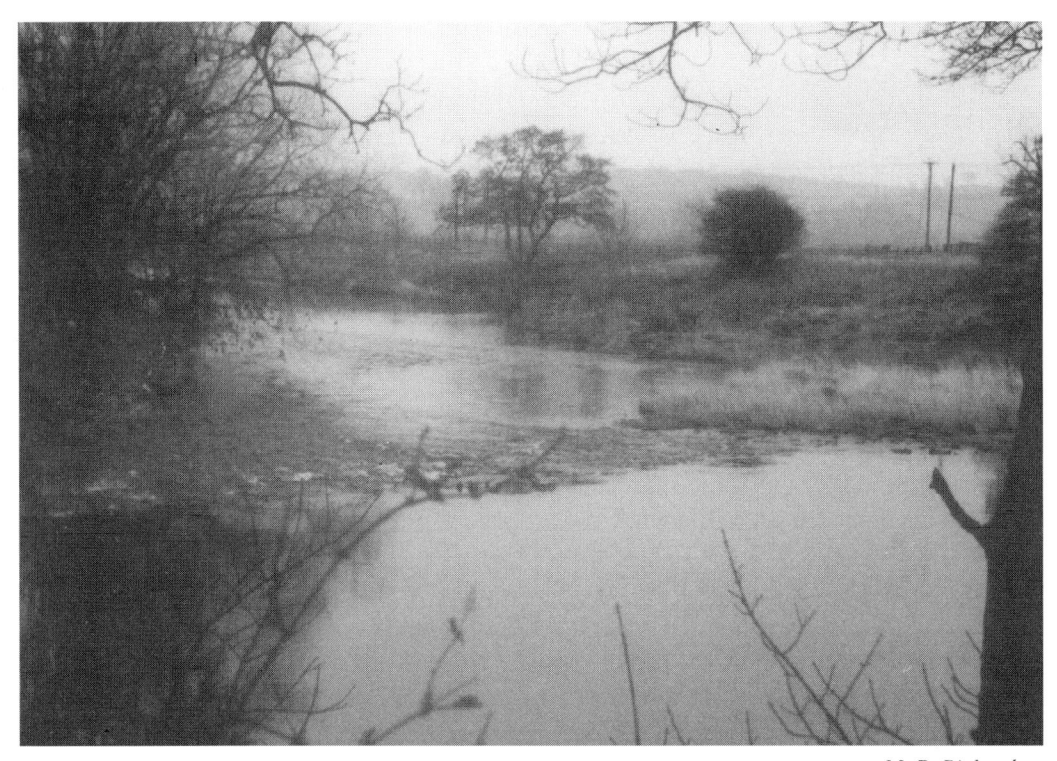

*M. R. Richardson*

26b. The River Wear at Kepier looking downstream, 1994, showing line of mill dam; site of mill near bush top right.

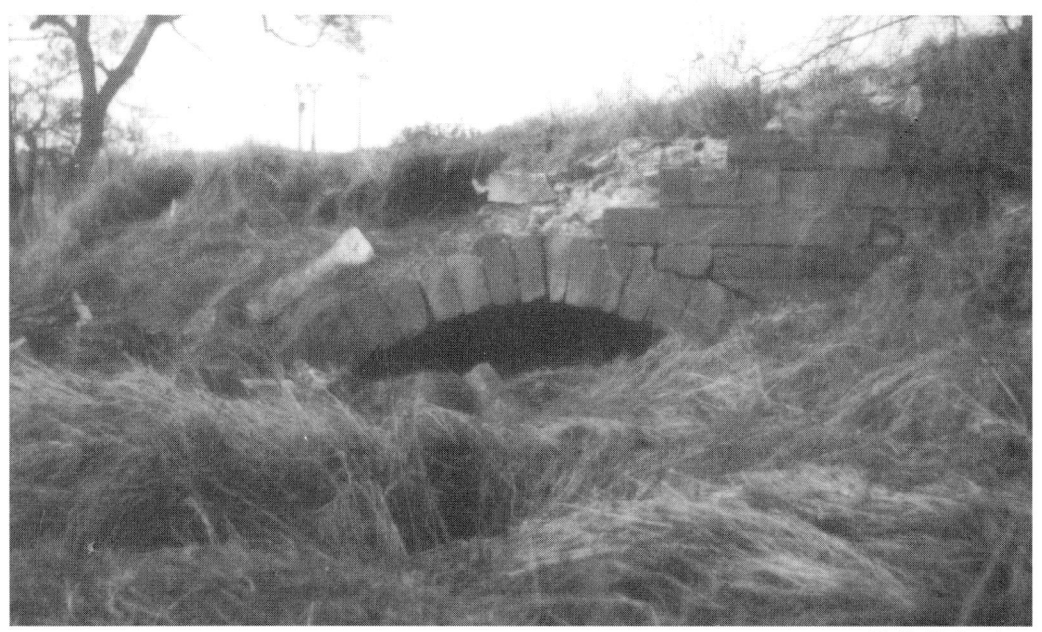

*M. R. Richardson*

27. Remains of arch of mill race.

## The last of the gardens and the inn

Kepier gardens continued to prosper during much of the nineteenth century. Surtees called them 'a summer place of public amusement' and The Durham Chronicle 'a favourite resort for the citizens of Durham and visitors from a distance.' So popular were they that a boat plied across the river bringing patrons who paid one penny for a return ticket. On Sundays especially the boat was crowded and the gardens 'were filled in every part.' An ordnance survey map of 1857 in the Londonderry Papers shows the laid-out gardens with walks between the beds, a path to a corner well and the orchard on the eastern slope.[107]

By this time the job of gardener was often linked with that of innkeeper of the White Bear and, in the early 1850s, with that of the miller as well. There was also a 'garden servant' lodging at the mill in 1851, according to the census returns of that year. No gardener is listed after 1871, although the name 'Kepier gardens' clung to the site until 1939. Ornamental plants and shrubs may have been sold and at length no sign of the gardens was left.[108]

Some of the last customers of the White Bear were members of the Society of Antiquaries of Newcastle-upon-Tyne. They arrived at Durham railway station on the afternoon of Saturday 21 September 1889 to visit St Giles' church and the chapel of St Mary Magdalen. Afterwards they walked by a field path to Kepier where they inspected the gateway and the old inn. Inside the latter they went into several rooms with carved oak panelling, noting that it was rather dilapidated. They partook of tea there before catching their train home at the end of a very pleasant afternoon.[109]

The decline in the prosperity of the area meant that fewer and fewer people had reason to walk out to Kepier. This affected trade at the inn and eventually it closed; it does not appear in the Durham Directory after 1891 and is recorded as being uninhabited in the Census returns for that year (completed 13 April). A correspondent of The Durham County Advertiser, 22 May 1891, lamented the neglect of the building. In a letter, signed 'Samuel Pickwick', he begged 'to draw the attention of our Archaeological Society to Kepier Hospital, which must be suffering from the weather driving in through the broken window casements.' Neither the learned body nor any individual responded to this plea and, in 1892, Sir Richard Musgrave ordered the inn to be dismantled.[110] It is said that the panelling and staircase were removed to a house in South Shields but this has not been traced.[111] All that remains today is the ground-floor arcade with some courses of brickwork and it is in a very unsound state. 'Within County Durham the building ranks as one of the most architecturally significant for its period of construction.' It is deserving of consolidation in the interests of safety so that detailed study can take place.[112]

## Lepers ?

In 1905 A.F. Leach, in his piece about Gilpin's school at Houghton, referred to the hospital at Kepier as having been for lepers. Mr. Leach must have picked up this information from those living in the neighbourhood, for it was thought to be true by many local people. An old man called Jack (b.1907) told of a time when he and other lads used to play in

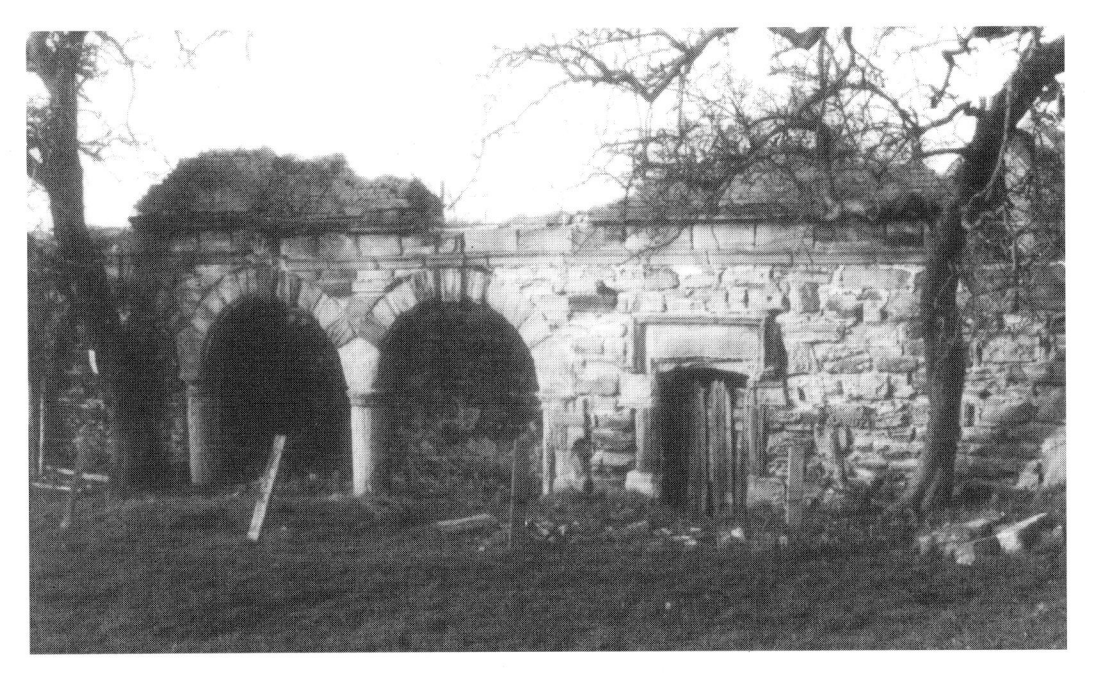

28a. Remains of the mansion house today. The two pear trees were drawn by Footitt and have grown unhindered during the hundred years since then.

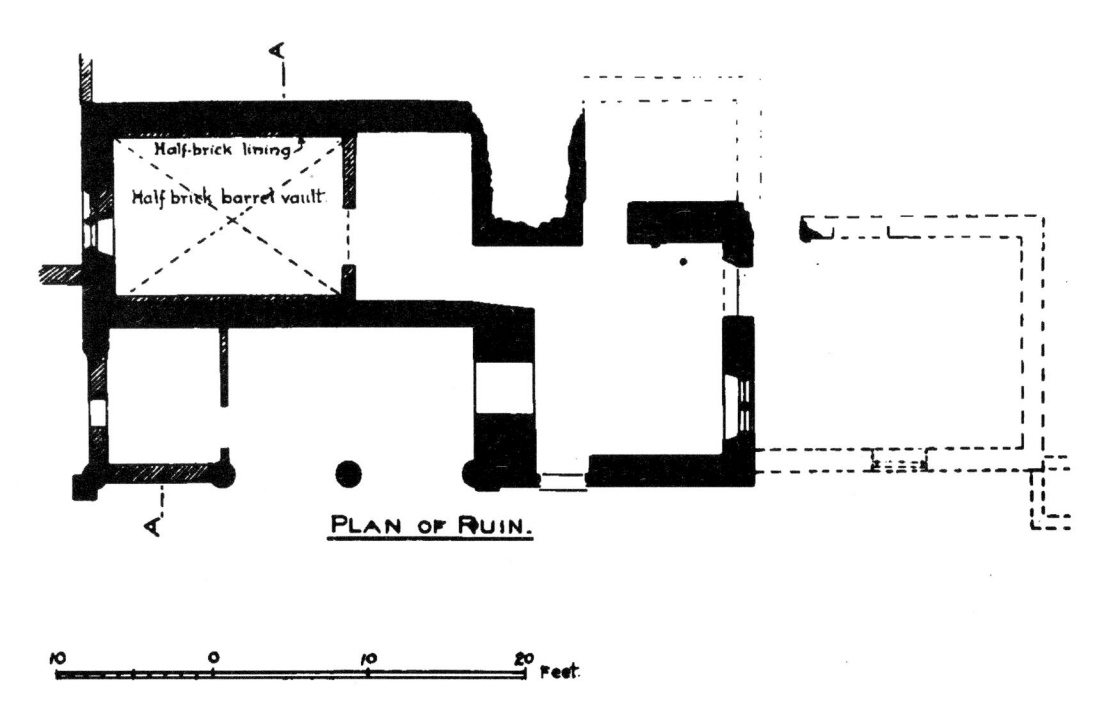

*W. G. Footitt*

28b. Plan of ruin of mansion house, 1917.

'the leper hospital, Harper's farm'. They would go into the blacksmith's shop and pull the bellows, until one of them shouted, 'You'll get leprosy!' at which they all ran out as fast as they could. There is nothing in the records about lepers at Kepier. Sherburn, a couple of miles away, could accommodate 65 lepers (although this changed in 1434 to the maintenance of 13 poor men and only two lepers, 'if so many could be found').[113]

Another leper hospital so close by was not needed. Indeed bishops and royalty would not have stayed at Kepier if there had been any danger of catching the dreaded disease.

### The North Eastern Electricity Board

Without the mill, the gardens and the inn, Kepier was left to tenant-farmers. Thomas Harper came in 1888 and was succeeded by his son, Robert, in 1908. Harrison Watson took over the farm on 1 May 1932 and a decade later had the unsettling experience of a change of ownership which threatened his tenancy.

Because of the run-down condition of the Kepier estate Sir Nigel Courtenay Musgrave tried to sell it in 1913 and again in 1918, without success. The North Eastern Electricity Board bought it on 27 October 1941 and, in 1944, announced its intention of building a large power station with 13 cooling towers on the fields beyond the gatehouse. The disastrous impact that this would have had on the landscape and the environment led the City of Durham Preservation Society (founded 1942, now the City of Durham Trust) to resist the scheme. It was joined by The Times and other national newspapers which took up the cause. So strong was the opposition that the Electricity Board gave up the project and the power station was built at Dunston on the Tyne instead. Kepier was sold on 25 June 1956 to Mr. Watson, then the tenant-farmer, and on his death in 1967 it passed to his daughter, Mrs. Ruth Watson, the present owner.[114]


## 21. AN END IN TRANQUILITY

Today Kepier lies in a byway of history. Strangers who wander along the riverside will be surprised to come across the great gateway, quite as big as that in the Bailey which once led to the cathedral priory. There is little within to tell them of former occupants - the aged local men for whom it was built, the influential masters and lordly bishops, a king and a queen, the Tudor incomers, Jacobean gentlemen and the people of the town who strolled out to the pleasure gardens. Now the place slumbers in an atmosphere of rural calm with only a few architectural remains and crumbling stones to indicate a more illustrious past.

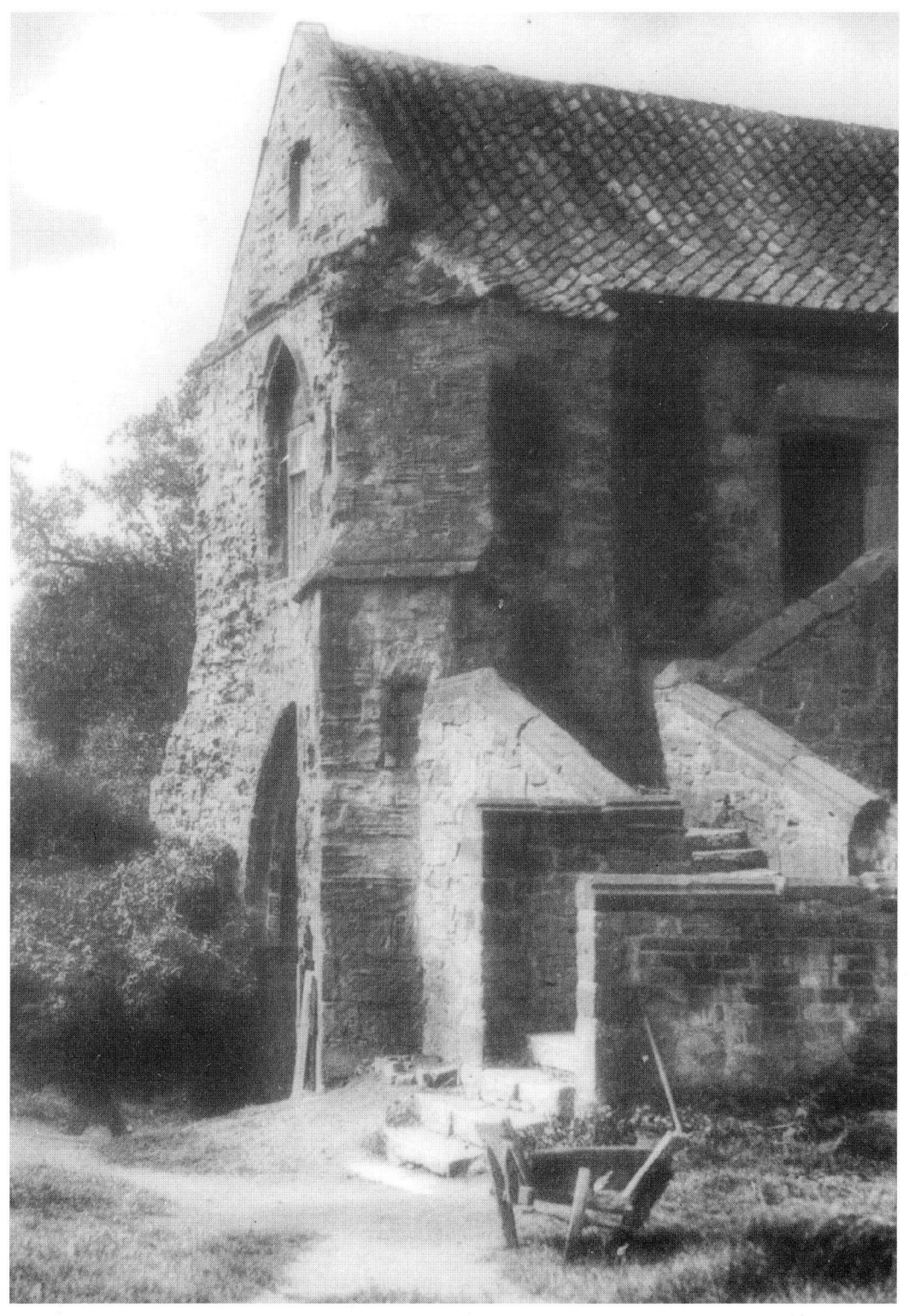

*Old photograph*

29. Rural retreat. East side of the gate-house from the north-east, late 1920s/early 1930s.

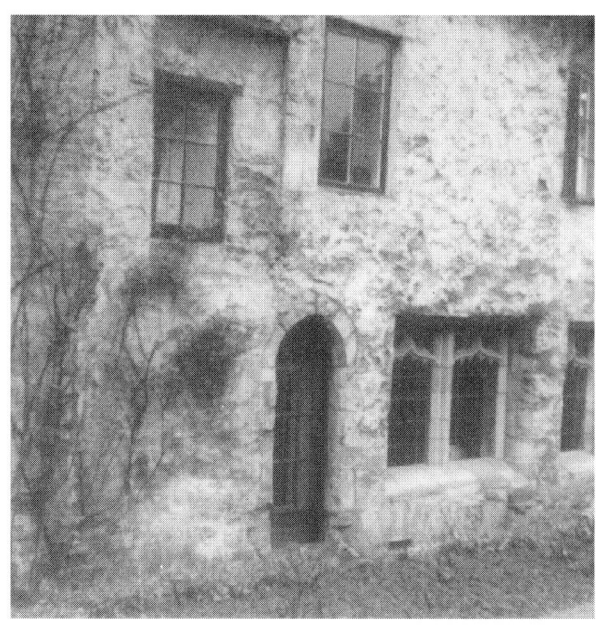

30a. Kepier Farm: east side, south end.
The door, shown blocked in Footitt's drawing (12), was re-opened in the 1950s. The window of two lights to its north side has fine tracery newly carved in the 1950s by Harold Jopling of Shincliffe, a Cathedral stone mason, to replace what had been removed earlier.

*Margaret Allen*

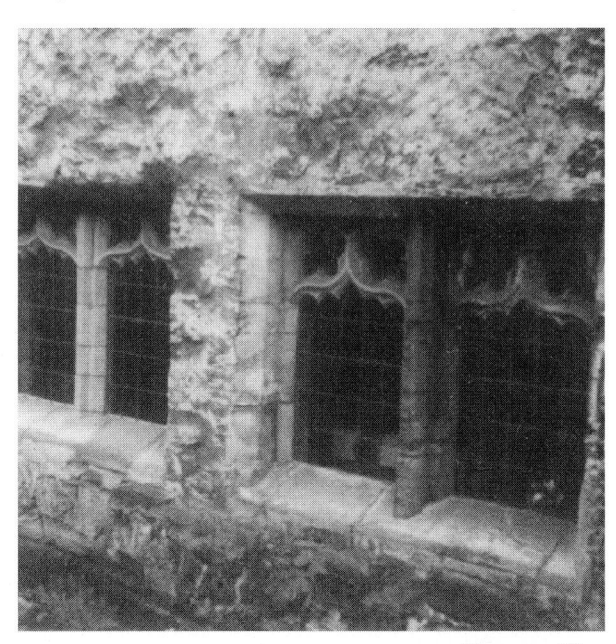

30b. Kepier Farm: east side, north end.
The tracery of the left light and half the second light buried in the east wall until the 1950s, was uncovered and renovated (at the same time as that on the south window) and is original.

*Margaret Allen*

Both 30a and 30b should be compared with the drawing by W. G. Footitt (12, page 23) where the northernmost of the east facing windows is shown with three lights. The one to the south has the left light and half the second blocked while the original tracery is visible in the remainder. The stone of a Tudor-style window was removed from the ruin of the Heath mansion and inserted in the south end of the farm house in the late 1940s.

# APPENDIX

## Notes on Illustrations

Front cover: Kepier Gatehouse today, photograph by Caroline Claughton

Inside Front Cover: Pedigree of Heath of Kepier, based on those in Surtees IV(II), 70, and C. R. Everett and C. Masterman, *The Pedigree of the Heath Family of Kepyer* ... (1914), Tables A and B.

Frontispiece: Fading Grandeur. Etching of west side of Kepier Gatehouse by H. Lea. Late 19th/early 20th century. Original owned by D. M. Meade.

1. Plan showing the location of Kepier Farm, Durham.

2. St Giles' church, Durham, by S. H. Grimm, 1777-84 *(British Library Board)*. The nave north wall with two small, round-headed windows is of Flambard's hospital chapel. It was heightened later, probably in the 15th century, together with the tower. The chancel was added about 1180, after the move to Kepier; the priest's doorway belongs there and not in the nave.

3. Seal of Kepier hospital, 1335, showing St Giles in mass vestments, holding a crosier in his left hand and a book in his right, with the hind looking up at him. Reproduced from *Memorials of St Giles* (Surtees Society, 95).

4. Tithe barn before demolition, 1964. It suffered from structural defects caused by mining subsidence. The asbestos sheeting on the roof replaced (after a fire) sandstone tiles fastened on with oak pegs. There was a tie beam roof system.

5. Plan and elevations of the tithe barn, High Grange, before 1964. The square joist holes indicate an earlier second floor. The triangular shapes, formed by sandstone slabs, are ventilation windows. *Transactions D. & N.* (NS I, 1968), 56.

6. Ruined chapel of the hospital of St Mary Magdalen, rebuilt in the 15th century, drawn by R. W. Billings, 1846. It remains in much the same condition today, but without the tracery of the east window, and can be seen near the Gilesgate roundabout.

7. Plan of Kepier Farm site, by Robin Taylor-Wilson.

8. Kepier hospital, drawn and enlarged by Martin Roberts, from Map of Durham City by Christopher Schwyzer, 1595 *(British Library Board)*.

9. West (outer) side of Kepier gateway (1333-45), by R. W. Billings, *Illustrations,* 1846. The line of quatrefoils over the arch (now partly

crumbled away) was then complete. The two shields above this were already eroded; Billings has imagined that the left one shows a face.

10. Shields above the front of Kepier gateway (now indecipherable). According to W. H. D. Longstaffe, the shield on the left *(azure, three crowns or)* attributed to St Edmund of Bury - was here used by Bishop Richard of Bury, during whose episcopate the gateway was built. C. H. Hunter Blair thought that the shield ought to have had an arrow through or between the crowns. (C. H. Hunter Blair (ed.), *Monuments in County Durham* (Newcastle upon Tyne Record Series, V, 1925), 119-20.) The shield on the right bore the arms of Edmund Howard *(gules, a bend argent between six cross crosslets of the same)*, master of the hospital at the time. The coats of arms would be coloured originally, giving the gateway a magnificent appearance.

11. Carvings on corbels supporting archway vault (a) crab-like creature, west end of south side, (b) frog-like creature, west end of north side. These would have been coloured originally. Permission for photography was kindly given by Mrs Ruth Watson.

12. Kepier farmhouse, facing east, by W. G. Footitt, an architect who lived nearby in Providence Row, June 1917. (Gibby Negative K13. Reproduced by permission of Durham University Library.) It depicts a 14th-century building with evidence of later alteration, especially to windows. The use as a farmhouse seems to date from at least the late 19th century.

13. East (inner) side of Kepier gateway and the attached buildings, by S. H. Grimm *(British Library Board)*. The 14th-century entrance on the north side of the arch gave access to the room above. The later steps and doorway to the upper floor were added by the Heaths. The medieval timber-framing of the west row is now covered externally but visible within.

14. A much-weathered crucifixion, flanked by St Mary and St John, now built into the west wall of the farmhouse, and probably originally in the chapel.

15. Carved head of a 15th-century man, probably a corbel, found when a trench for a water-main was dug in the orchard in 1961. The curled hair slants up from the nape of the neck, the brow is covered by a fringe and there is a moustache. A small cap is worn. Perhaps the carving represents a wealthy donor. A similar head was found among a load of stones from Kepier in the early 1960s and now graces the porch of a modern house. The present owner of Kepier remembers stone from a demolished pig-sty being sold at that time. The heads would be coloured originally.

16. Arms, crest and motto (trans. 'I hope for better things') of Heath of Kepier (coat of arms after C. R. Everett & C. Masterman, *op.cit.*, Table A.), granted 4 August 1558. An example of the arms appears on the wooden chest bearing the effigy of John Heath (d.1590), in St Giles' church, although the gold and black have been transposed.

17. Inscription on the west wall of Kepier school-house, Houghton-le-Spring. The house is dated by Pevsner as probably of 1724. This stone was seen by Surtees (Vol. I, 162), who says it 'records some considerable repairs and additions, made in 1779, at the expense of John Tempest of Wynyard'. This patron was one of the governors and a descendant of John Heath (see illustration 19).

The Latin text and translation are given below:

*Munificentia*
*Johannis Tempest, Arm.*
*XMDCCLXXIX*

*By the munificence of*
*John Tempest, Armiger*
*1779*

18. Inscription over the door of Kepier School, Houghton-le-Spring. The initials in the last line but one refer to Christopher Hunter, M.B., a former pupil (b.1695) and well-known antiquary, who placed it here.

The Latin text, seen by both Hutchinson (Vol.II, 1787, 561) and Surtees (Vol.I, 1816, 162) is given below with free translation.

*Schola de Keepier*
*Ab Eliz. Angliae Regina*
*Ao MDLXXIV. Fundata*
*Ex Procuratione I. Heath, Ar.*
*Et B. Gilpin, Rect. Eccl. Houghto.*
*C. H. M. B. Alumnus Posuit*
*Ao MDCCXXIV*

*The Kepier School, founded in the year 1574 by Elizabeth, Queen of England, through the zeal of John Heath, Armiger, and Bernard Gilpin, Rector of the Church of Houghton. Christopher Hunter, Bachelor of Medicine, a former pupil, has placed this here, in the year 1724.*

19. Wooden effigy, supposed to represent John Heath of Kepier (d. 1590), represented in plate armour. The head lies on a tilting helmet with the

crest of a cock's head attached by a wreath. The feet rest on a scroll enfolding two death's heads; above and below these, respectively, are inscribed the words, HODIE MICHI and CRAS TIBI ('Today is mine, tomorrow thine').

Both Hutchinson (Vol.II, 303) and Surtees (Vol.IV, pt. 2, 58) describe the crest as a bear's paw, 'not the usual crest of Heath'. When Boyle wrote in 1892 the crest had become the cock's head of Heath. T. Nicholson, in The Heath Family of Kepier ( see note 80), 55-6, repeats a theory that the effigy was originally intended for another person and was not given a Heath cognizance until sometime between 1840 and 1892.

20. The Kepier site from the east by S. H. Grimm *(British Library Board)* showing, left to right, the earliest-known sketch of the Heath mansion house, the gatehouse, the timber-framed west row and the building used as the farmhouse.

21. The Heath mansion, 1883-8, when Thomas Anderson was the innkeeper. South and west elevations drawn by W. G. Footitt (Gibby Negative K14b. Reproduced by permission of Durham University Library). Some original leaded panes then survived. The ground-floor window (west side) is the same one photographed in illustration 27. The stonework of the loggia is in good condition, with its keystone patterns and shields showing clearly. The west-facing and a south-facing arch are blocked up. An eastern extension, apparently of the late 18th century has replaced a smaller original annex ( *see illustration* 20).

22. Layout of the Kepier garden as shown in the Ordnance Survey of 1858. The small square and rectangle near the west boundary wall probably represent summer-houses. The pear orchard on the east side slopes down towards the garden plots; several of these trees remain and in places the original lines of planting can be distinguished.

23. The Heath mansion from the north-west, by F. W. Morgan, *c.* 1887, sketch book 15 *(by courtesy of The British Architectural Library, RIBA, London)*. Thanks are due to Professor G. R. Batho and Mr M. F. Richardson for bringing the Morgan sketch books to my notice.

24. Bricked-up gateway to the Heath mansion grounds. It should be compared with the Morgan drawing which shows that it was already bricked up in 1887.

25. Filled-in window in west wall of the Heath mansion. Already blocked

when Morgan did his sketch, the central mullion, there shown, has since been removed.

26a. Kepier panorama, showing (left to right) the ruins of the mill, the gate-house with attached row of buildings, the roof of the farmhouse and the Heath mansion (Kepier or White Bear Inn). The line of the mill dam, with some stakes remaining, is evident and may be compared with the line of the weir marked on illustration 24. Dated 1870-92.

26b. River Wear at Kepier looking downstream, 1994, line of mill dam still clearly showing. Site of mill is near the bush, top right. Off picture, right, is the hospital gateway.

27. All that is left of Kepier mill (1988), burned down in 1870, is the arch through which the mill race once flowed. Its position at the base of the building can be discerned in the previous illustration.

28a. Plan of ruin of mansion house, measured and drawn by W. G. Footitt, September 1917. (Gibby Negative K14b. Reproduced by permission of Durham University Library.)

28b. Remains of the mansion house today. The two pear trees were drawn by Footitt (Crosby, *Old Photographs* ) and have grown unhindered during the hundred years since then.

29. Rural retreat. East side of the gate-house from the north-east, late 1920s/early 1930s. (Collection of M. F. Richardson.)

30a & b. Harold Jopling's fine work may be seen in Durham Cathedral, especially in the Neville Screen where the second pinnacle from the north is his copy of the original which was badly decayed.

Inside Back Cover: Pedigree of Cole of Gateshead, Kepier and Brancepeth. Based on pedigree in Brancepeth Estate catalogue, Vol. I *(Durham County Record office)*.

Back Cover: Water-colour of the west side of Kepier gatehouse (1774-5) by William Beilby. The small close adjoining on the right has pear trees espaliered against the inner wall. The entrance from the garden was bricked up in the 1950s.

# ABBREVIATIONS

| | |
|---|---|
| AA | *Archaeologia Aeliana* |
| APC | *Acts of the Privy Council* |
| A.S.C. | Durham University Library Archives and Special Collections |
| Billings, *Illustrations* | R.W. Billings, *Illustrations of the Architectural Antiquities of the County of Durham* (London, 1846) |
| Boyle | J.R. Boyle, *Comprehensive Guide to the County of Durham* (Walter Scott, Ltd., London, 1892). |
| BRUC | A.B. Emden, *A Biographical Register of the University of Cambridge to A.D. 1500* (C.U.P., 1963) |
| BRUO | A.B. Emden, *A Biographical Register of the University of Oxford to A.D. 1500,* (O.U.P., 1957). |
| CPR | *Calendar of the Patent Rolls* |
| CUP | Cambridge University Press |
| DD | *The Durham Directory and Almanack* (George Walker, Jun.,Durham, 1847-1916) |
| DCYB | *Durham City Year Book . . . ,* 1922-53. |
| DNB | *Dictionary of National Biography* |
| DRO | Durham Record Office |
| *Fasti* | *Fasti Dunelmenses* (ed. D.S. Boutflower, SS 139, 1926) |
| Hutchinson | W. Hutchinson, *The History and Antiquities of the County Palatine of Durham*, 3 vols (Newcastle, 1785, 1787, and 1794) |
| LP | *Letters and Papers, Foreign and Domestic, of the Reign of Henry VIII*, XX, XXI (ed. J. Gairdner and R.H. Brodie, 1905-10) |
| *Memorials* | *Memorials of St Giles's, Durham,* (ed. J. Barmby, SS 95, 1895) |
| NS | New series |
| OUP | Oxford University Press |
| Pevsner | N. Pevsner, *The Buildings of England: County Durham* (Harmondsworth, Penguin Books, 1953, rev. 1983). |
| *PSA (Newcastle)* | *Proceedings of the Society of Antiquaries of Newcastle-upon-Tyne* |
| *Reg Pal Dun* | *Registrum Palatinum Dunelmense*, I-IV, (ed. T. DuffusHardy, 1873-8) |
| *Scrip Tres* | *Historiae Dunelmensis Scriptores Tres* (ed. J. Raine, SS 9, 1839) |
| Surtees | R. Surtees, *The History and Antiquities of the County* |

|  |  |
|---|---|
|  | *Palatine of Durham*, I-IV (1816-40) |
| SS | Surtees Society |
| Taylor-Wilson | A Report on the Preliminary Building Survey of John Heath's 'Kepier House' at Kepier Farm, Durham, by Robin Taylor-Wilson (Department of Archaeology, University of Durham, 1993, unpublished). |
| *Test Ebor* | *Testamenta Eboracensia*, I, III, V, ed. J. Raine, SS 4 (1836), 45 (1864) and 79 (1884). |
| *Trans D & N* | *Transactions of the Architectural and Archaeological Society of Durham and Northumberland.* |
| *Valor* | *Valor Ecclesiasticus Tempore Henrici* VIII, I-VI (ed. J. Caley and J. Hunter, Record Commission, 1810-34). |
| *VCH Durham* | *The Victoria County History of Durham,* I-III (ed. W. Page, London, 1905, 1907, 1928). |
| *Wills* | *Wills and Inventories . . .*, I, II, IV, ed. J. Raine, SS 2(1835), 38 (1860) and 142 (1929). |

# Documents in Durham County Record Office

|  |  |
|---|---|
| D/Lo | Londonderry Estate Papers (reproduced by permission of the Marquess of Londonderry and the County Archivist). |
| D/Lo/D 47 | Abstracts from Gilesgate Court Rolls (1518-56) |
| D/Lo/F 270 | Marriage settlement of John Tempest and Elizabeth Heath, 1642 |
| D/Lo/F 320 | Settlement to secure jointure on Dorothy Heath, 1630 |
| D/Lo/F 321 | Conveyance to secure an annuity to Margery Craddock, 1648 |
| D/Lo/P 75 | Ordnance Survey plan, 1959 (by permission also of the Ordnance Survey) |
| D/X 790/1 | Records of the Manor Court of Gilligate, vol. I (from 1534) |

# Notes

Notes already given in D.M. Meade, 'The Hospital of Saint Giles at Kepier, near Durham, 1112-1545', and 'The Medieval Parish of Saint Giles, Durham', in *Trans. D & N*, NS I (1968) and II (1970), respectively, are not repeated here.

1. J. Sumption, *Pilgrimage* (Faber & Faber, London, 1975), 116-7.
2. Peter F. Ryder, St Giles' Church, Durham: An Archaeological Assessment (Unpublished report for the Diocese of Durham, October 1991), 9.
3. R.M. Clay, *The Mediaeval Hospitals of England* (Methuen, London, 1909; reprinted F. Cass, 1966), 149, 158; Surtees, IV (II), 149.
4. R.M. Clay, *op.cit.*, 157, 162; R.B. Dobson, *Durham Priory, 1400-1450* (CUP 1973), 169.
5. Even earlier, in February 1302/03, the working centre is recorded as being called 'Caldecote grange' and, in 1323, as 'the grange of Caldecotes', see M.M. Camsell, 'Development of a Northern Town in the Later Middle Ages', II (b) (unpublished D.Phil. thesis, York, 1985), 467, 470.
6. M. Bonney, *Lordship and the Urban Community* (Cambridge University Press, 1990), 55. By the late thirteenth century this mill was in the possession of the almoner and it remained in use throughout the medieval period. It 'only ceased to be used as a mill within living memory', VCH *Durham*, II, 64.
7. H.S. Offler (ed.), *Durham Episcopal Charters, 1071-1152* (SS 179, 1968), 64-7. The 15 villages were Newbottle, Houghton [-le-Spring], Wearmouth, Ryhope, Easington, Sedgefield, Sherburn, Quarrington, Newton [by Durham], Chester[-le-Street], Washington, Boldon, Cleadon, Whickham, and Ryton. For thraves, see Section 5, Puiset's endowments.
8. According to the Rule of St Benedict, R.M. Clay, *op.cit.*, 3.
9. R.C. Finucane, *Miracles and Pilgrims* (Dent, London, 1977), 126-7.
10. A. Young, *William Cumin: Border Politics and the Bishopric of Durham, 1141-1144* (Borthwick Papers, no. 54, 1978), 1, 10, 11, 21-5; *The Chronicle of John, Prior of Hexham*, trans. J. Stevenson, in series *The Church Historians of England* (Seeleys, London), IV part I (1856), 18-23.
11. V.E. Watts, 'Some Northumbrian Fishery Names, I', in *Trans. D & N*, NS 6 (1982), 89. C.W. Gibby, *Sherburn Hospital, Durham* (c.1977), 4. Salmon were witnessed running up the river to spawn some 700 years after the refoundation. Police Constable Joseph Scott said, 'There were hundreds of fine salmon fish at the place [Kepier Mill] at the time [about 8.30 p.m., on Friday 11 October 1867] in question.' *The Durham Chronicle*, 18 October 1867.
12. G.A.L. Johnson and Kingsley Dunham, 'The Stones of Durham Cathedral: A Preliminary Note', in *Trans., D & N*, NS 6 (1982), 53, 54.

13. This word was used for lay-brothers by the Cistercian Order and was possibly inserted here by mistake, instead of *fratri*. Puiset was a friend to the Cistercians and the word may have been known in Durham without being properly understood by the clerk who wrote out Puiset's regulations. (I am indebted to Mrs. Jean Scammell for this explanation.) See also G.V. Scammell, *Hugh du Puiset* (CUP, 1956), 107-9.
14. Thirteen was a favourite number, being reminiscent of Christ and his disciples, see Clay, *op.cit.*, 145.
    In 1316 King Edward II sent a mandate to the 'brethren and sisters' of the hospital; and 'sisters' were mentioned again by Bishop Tunstall in 1532. There were never any women on the Kepier staff, so these references must have been slips on the part of the clerks or else the use of a formal phrase. See *VCH Durham*, II, 112.
15. H.S. Offler, *op.cit.*, 66-7.
16. *Memorials*, 199; Ryder, op.cit., 9; R.M. Clay, *op.cit.*, 111-5.
17. J. Barmby (ed.), *Memorials*, Frontispiece (illustrations), 269-70 (description); *Catalogue of the Seals in the Treasury of the Dean and Chapter of Durham.* From a manuscript made by W. Greenwell. Collated and annotated by C.H.H. Blair (1911-21), VIII, Durham Seals, xlviii-ix, 149-50; W.H.D. Longstaffe, 'The Banner and Cross of Saint Cuthbert', in AA, NS II (1858), 56-7.
18. But, at a general array of the clergy on Gilesgate Moor on 24 March 1399/1400, preparatory to Henry IV's expedition into Scotland, the master of Kepier attended with one lancer and two archers. See *Scrip Tres*, Appendix CLXII, clxxxv.
19. M. Bonney, *op.cit.*, 48-9; K.E. Bayley (ed.), 'Two thirteenth-century assize rolls for the County of Durham', in *Miscellanea* II (SS 127, 1916), no. 294; *Memorials*, 168.
20. C.M. Fraser (ed.) *Durham Quarter Sessions Rolls*, 1471-1625 (SS 199, 1991), 280, 293. The bishop's bakehouse (i.e. for the use of the people in the bishop's borough) was in Walkergate (also Bakehouse Lane, also Back Lane). It was still so-called in 1748, although by 1766 it was referred to as 'the common bakehouse.' McKay and Sons, Ltd. (Carpet Factory) records DRO D/Ma 12, deeds dated 2 October 1748, 20 October 1766 and 11 May 1792.
21. J.E. Parsons, 'Kepier Tithe Barn', in *Trans*. D & N, NS I (1968), 56, 57. The only mention of the tithe barn found is in a settlement of property, 1629/30, D/Lo/F 320. The 'seat house [i.e. mansion house] wherein Thomas Snawdon dwelleth and the great barn there only excepted', refers to the house and tithe barn at West Grange. Thomas Snawdon was recorded as being tenant of Hither [or West] Grange in 1644: R. Welford (ed.), *Royalist Compositions in Durham and Northumberland* (SS 111, 1905), 20.

22. M. Bonney, *op.cit.*, 100-1; *Memorials,* 18 note 1.
23. M. Bonney, *op.cit.*, 198, 216-7, 223-4. For court records see DRO D/Lo/D47, DRO D/X 790/1 and *Memorials*, 163-8.
24. M. Bonney, *op.cit.*, 181; M.M. Camsell, op.cit., 426-7, 432, 460, 484.
25. *Memorials,* xxii, xxix-xxxiii, 206; H.S. Offler, op.cit., 170-2; Surtees, IV (11), 67-8: *VCH Durham*, II, 119-20.
26. J. Stevenson (ed.), *Libellus de Vita et Miraculis Sancti Godrici* (SS 20, 1845), 143 and note 3.
27. J.T. Fowler (ed.), *Durham Account Rolls*, I (SS 99, 1898), 225, 240; R.B. Dobson, *op.cit.,* 168.
28. J.T. Fowler, *op.cit.*, 228 (wedding), 230 (parish), 240 (font), 253 (burial).
29. C.M. Fraser (ed.), *Records of Antony Bek* (SS 162, 153), 178-9; *Reg Pal Dun*, I, index under 'Kypier, letters dated at'; J. Raine (ed.), *Depositions . . . and other Ecclesiastical Proceedings from the Court of Durham* (SS 21, 1845), 8-9.
30. *Reg Pal Dun*, III, lxxxii, 122-3. The title 'of Bisaccia [Italy]' is a nominal one. This suffragan is known to have been in the Durham diocese 1342-5.
31. List of Records of Kepier School and Almshouse, Houghton-le-Spring, made by Martin Snape, Items No. 24 and No. 25, held at Durham Record Office; C.M. Fraser, *A History of Antony Bek,* (1957), 47 and n.4, 232; *Fasti*, 52, 61.
32. In spite of this, the master was summoned to attend a synod in the Galilee chapel of the cathedral on 4 October 1507, see *Scrip Tres*, Appendix CCCXVI, cccciv.
33. In 1321 these tithes, with others at Gateshead, were commuted for a payment of four marks (£2-66) at Pentecost and Martinmas, see *Memorials*, xxvii note 1.
34. Billings, *Illustrations*, two sketches at end of volume; C.H. Hunter Blair (ed.), *Monuments in County Durham* (Newcastle upon Tyne Record Series, V, 1925), 119-20, re shields on west front of gateway; Boyle, 389; Johnson and Dunham, *op.cit.*, 54 and Figure 1; Pevsner, *County Durham*, 255-6; PSA *(Newcastle),* NS IV, no. 12 (1889), 139, account of visit to Kepier (W.H.D. Longstaffe's opinion on the shields quoted); Taylor-Wilson, Figure 2; *VCH Durham,* III, 183-4; map of Durham City by Christopher Schwyzer, 1595. I am grateful to Mr Martin Roberts for pointing out a medieval doorway within the ruined Heath house, east side; for his opinion on the buildings north of the gatehouse; and for allowing me to use his notes on the gatehouse roof (the detailed results of his investigations here will appear as a future report of the North East Vernacular Architecture Group).
35. G.W. Kitchin (ed.), *Richard d'Aungerville of Bury. Fragments of his Register and other Documents* (SS 119, 1910), 104 and starred note; *Memorials*, xxvii-viii, 215-22; Surtees, IV (II), 64; VCH *Durham,* II, 113.

36. C.C. Bishopric, Clerk of Works account, 190045, m.3. The Kepier entry in this document, and its significance, was pointed out to me by Mrs Linda Drury.
37. *Memorials*, 252.
38. *Fasti*, 78.
39. *BRUO*, 918.
40. *Test Ebor*, I, 405. Wyclif's armorial bearings (argent, a chevron sable between three cross crosslets gules) can be seen on the roof of the west alley of the cathedral cloisters (see *Memorials, 257* note).
41. *Fasti*, 43, 89; *Memorials*, 254 and note 1; *Reg Pal Dun*, IV, 144; *VCH Durham*, II, 112-3; C.M. Fraser (ed.), *Northern Petitions* (SS 194, 1981), 189-90.
42. *Memorials*, 224-7; *Scrip Tres*, Appendix CCXI, ccxliii-vii; R.L. Storey, *Thomas Langley and the Bishopric of Durham, 1406-1437* (S.P.C.K., London, 1961), 79, 192; *VCH Durham*, II, 113.
43. G. Hinde (ed.), *The Registers of Cuthbert Tunstall, Bishop of Durham, 1530-59. . . .* (SS 161, 1952), 22-3; *VCH Durham*, II, 113. An almost identical notice was sent to Greatham in September.
44. *Test Ebor*, I, 403-5 (Inventory); J. Raine (ed.) *Wills*, I, 66-8; *Memorials, 257* note.
45. *BRUC*, 79; *Scrip Tres*, Appendix CCCI, ccclxxxvii-viii; *Test Ebor*, III (SS 45, 1865), 250 double-starred note.
46. *Fasti*, 51; *Memorials*, 259 note 1; *Test Ebor*, III, 281 double-crossed note, 282 starred note. According to his will, dated 8 February 1482/83, Gillow wished to be buried in Houghton-le-Spring church, of which he was rector, near to his mother. He provided for a chantry chapel to be erected over his body and this can be seen as a detached structure (connected by a passage) on the south side of the chancel, now used as a vestry.
47. *BRUC*, 367.
48. This list is taken from the *VCH Durham*, II, 113, but amended from other sources, as follows:
C.M. Fraser, 'Officers of Durham under Antony Bek', in AA, Fourth series, xxxv (1957), 25-6, for Peter de Thoresby; *BRUC*, 79, for Ralph Booth, and 367, for Roger Layborn; *BRUO*, 918, for Hugh Herle, and 1164-5, DNB, for William Franklyn; *Fasti*, 89, for Hugh de Monte Alto, 78, for William Legat, 146, for Thomas Wytton, and 16, for John Boer; Greenslade, S.L., 'The site of St John's College, Durham, 1541-1800', in *Durham Johnian*, No.2 (January 1948), 6-10; and 'Towards the mediaeval history of the site of St John's College, Durham', in *Durham Johnian*, No.3 (January 1949), pp. 22-6; for John Lound (Greenslade has 1467 for Lound's termination of office, but in ASC Frosterley Manor Records 28 p. 253 Henry Gillow appears as master on 25 June 1465); M.P. Howden (ed.), *The Register of Richard Fox, Lord Bishop of Durham, 1494-1501* (SS,

147, 1932), 50, for Ralph Booth and Thomas Colston, also 165-6 for Thomas Colston and Roger Layborn; A.S.C: Frosterley Manor Records 28, Manor of Frosterley Court Book, 1465-1808, 253, for Henry Gillow. Meldred is inserted although he was in office before the move to Kepier. *Memorials* has interesting footnotes on some of the masters.

49. *Valor,* V, 307-8; C. Sturge, *Cuthbert Tunstal* (Longmans, Green and Co., London, 1938), 199 and notes 1 and 2.

50. J.J. Vickerstaff, *A Great Revolutionary Deluge? Education and the Reformation in County Durham* (Teesside Paper in North Eastern History, No.2, University of Teesside, 1992), 15-16.

51. A.S.C., Frosterley Court Book, 28, 1.

52. G. Baskerville, *English Monks and the Suppression of the Monasteries* (Bedford Historical Series, 7, London, 1937), 58-9. Sir John also acted in a similar capacity for the college of Staindrop, near Barnard Castle, and the priory of Guisborough in Yorkshire, his yearly fees being £1 6s. 8d. and £4 6s. 8d., respectively, *Valor,* V, 311, 81. For some details of the Bulmer family see the will of Sir William Bulmer, father of Sir John, in *Test Ebor*, V (SS 79, 1884), 306-13 and footnotes; also the will of Sir Ralph Bulmer, son of Sir John, in *North Country Wills*, II (SS 121, 1912), 7 and footnote.

53. Baskerville, *op.cit.,* 60-1. In his will John Franklyn left to his brother 'two drinking pots of silver which was my uncle's the dean of Windsor' (i.e. William Franklyn), *Wills,* I, 387.

54. Baskerville, *op.cit.,* 61.

55. *Alumni Cantabrigienses*, Pt I, vol. II (CUP, 1922), 176; DNB, under William Franklyn.

56. M. James, *Family, Lineage, and Civil Society* (Clarendon Press, Oxford, 1974), 8.

57. Hinde, *op.cit.,* 2. The annual income of Sherburn hospital was also £100 at this time (£142 0s 4d in 1535) and that of Greatham was £26 13s. 4d. (£34 13s. 4d.in 1535).

58. A.G. Dickens, *The English Reformation* (B.T. Batsford, Ltd., London, 1964, rev. edn., 1967), 77.

59. M.H. & R. Dodds, *The Pilgrimage of Grace*... 2 vols. (CUP, 1915), I, 203.

60. *Ibid,* I, 205, 237-8, 258; II, 24, 163-4, 214. Also on 25 May Sir John's wife, Margaret, was burned at Smithfield for supporting her husband and as an example to others, II, 215-6; *Memorials,* 167. Sir John and his wife are leading characters in H.F.M. Prescott's novel about the Pilgrimage of Grace, *The Man on a Donkey* (1952).

61. The second-named agent was probably James Rokeby, auditor of the Court of Augmentations in the bishopric of Durham,. See W.C. Richardson, *History of the Court of Augmentations* (Baton Rouge, Louisiana State University Press, 1961), 54 note 62; LP, xx(1), 27 no. 60 and 271 no. 557 (f.70).

62. Clay, *op.cit.*, 232.
63. Sturge, *op.cit.*, 261; LP, xx(1), 61 no. 131.
64. *LP*, xx(1), 122 no. 282 (14) and 77 no. 149(39). Paget sold the manor of Hunstanworth, including its rectory, to William Eccleston and Henry Doyle in November 1545, see *LP* xx(1), 77 no. 149 (39) and xx(2), 329 no. 52.
65. *BRUO, A.D. 1501 to 1540* (Oxford, 1974), 146-7; DNB, under Richard Cox; H.A. Doubleday and Lord Howard de Walden (ed.), *The Complete Peerage*, 4 (Alan Sutton, Gloucester, 1982), under Paget, 280 note f.
66. *LP*, xx(1), 461 no. 939.
67. For Richard Forester see *Wills*, I, 407-8; and St Nicholas' burial register, 1540-1603, 81 (DRO EP/Du.SN1/1); also S.L. Greenslade, 'The Last Monks of Durham Cathedral Priory', in *The Durham University Journal*, NS X, Vol. XL1 (1948-9), 109, 112. It is possible that Richard Forster transferred to the cathedral priory, for the last monk to enter there had the same name, taking priestly orders between June 1538 and September 1539. This monk was assigned a pension from the surrender of the Convent on 31 December 1539. If he had come from Kepier it is quite likely that he returned there (information from Mr Alan Piper); for Anthony Middleton see *Wills* II, 35-7; St Margaret's burial register, DRO EP/Du. M/1; Surtees IV (II), 146; and DRO D/Lo/D 47.
68. *LP*, xx(1), 76-7, no. 149 (39). Paget was elevated to the peerage as Lord Paget of Beaudesert [Staffordshire] in the reign of Edward VI, 3 December 1549. His descendants became (from 1815) Marquesses of Anglesey.
69. *LP*, xxi(2), 439 no. 774 (142).
70. *Fasti*, 53.
71. *Wills*, II, 4; J. Raine, *Depositions*, 137.
72. *Wills*, I, 386-91 (John Franklyn's will); A.S.C. Probate Register IVf 186v (John Blarton's will); Houghton-le-Spring burial register, DRO EP/HO 1.
73. *DNB* for William Franklyn.
74. Clay, *op.cit.*, 227.
75. A.S.C., Frosterley Court Book, 55.
76. *APC*, III, 388; IV, 31; V, 166, 206; Meade, 'St Giles', 67 and note 26, for marble cross (this cross is now shown to have been moved to the market place by 25 March 1555); M.H. Merriman, 'The Assured Scots'. in *The Scottish Historical Review*, 47 (1968), 23, 24, 25, 27, 33, 34; Sturge, *op.cit.*, 310; 'Short Statement of Title to the Rectory of St Giles', 1914 (on behalf of the Marquess of Londonderry), in the papers of the Gilligate Church Estate Charity, by permission of the Trustees: Bargain and Sale: John Cockburn to John Heath of London, Esq. of (int.al) the Rectories of St Nicholas and St Giles and all tithes, etc., 25 March 1555; Surtees IV (11), 65-6. The fine levied between John Heath and John Cockburn gave the authority of a court (1568) to the agreement made earlier (1555);

Thanks to Mrs Linda Drury for clarifying the apparent discrepancy in dating.

77. *The Inventories of Church Goods. . . .* (SS 97, 1896), 152.
78. *Memorials,* 168, 169; J. Foster, *Pedigrees recorded at the Visitations of the County Palatine of Durham* (Joseph Foster, London, 1887), 156, 157.
79. *CPR,* Elizabeth, I, 237; C.T. Clay, 'The Keepership of the Old Palace of Westminster', in *The English Historical Review* LIX (1944), 15; R.B. Pugh, *Imprisonment in Medieval England* (CUP, 1968), 119, 155, 158, 171-2; C.R. Everett and C. Masterman, *The Pedigree of the Heath Family of Kepyer . . . .* (M.S. Dodds, Newcastle-upon-Tyne, 1914), 9; Surtees IV (11), 66, 70, 71; *VCH Durham,* III, 185, and note 29. Evidence of John Heath's friendship with the clergy is contained in his will, whereby he left money to both Bishop Matthew Hutton, Dean Tobias Matthew and the latter's wife to buy them mourning rings. Also, the Dean was one of the overseers of the will.
80. *CPR,* Elizabeth, VI, 318; Enrolment of Inquisition Post Mortem, 27 August 1576, in 'Short Statement of Title. . . .', 1 (see note 74).
81. G. Battiscombe, *Bernard Gilpin* (The Gilpin Press, Houghton-le-Spring, 1947), 19-20, 22; *CPR,* Elizabeth, VI, 244 no. 1293; D. Marcombe, 'Bernard Gilpin: Anatomy of an Elizabethan Legend', in *Northern History* XVI (1980), 33-4; PSA *(Newcastle),* NS VIII (1899), 202; Surtees, I, 158, 159 and IV (II), 66, 71; *VCH Durham*, I, 393-6.
82. *Memorials,* 132 and note 2; Surtees IV (II), 66, 71.
83. R. Annis and P. Ryder, 'Bradley Hall', in *Archaeology North*, 4 (December 1992), 20, 21; Boyle, 389-90; T. Nicholson, 'The Heath Family of Kepyer', in *Antiquities of Sunderland and its vicinity*, xix (1929-32), 57; Taylor-Wilson, passim (unpaged). Espaliered trees in the west enclosure are shown on W. Beilby's water-colour (front cover). Mrs Ruth Watson informs me that there were stumps of old pear trees there when she first came to Kepier.
84. *Memorials,* 134; *Wills,* IV, 65-70.
85. DRO D/X 790/1, 1, 87.
86. Surtees, IV (II), 66 and note q; *VCH Durham*, III, 185.
87. DRO D/Lo/F 320.
88. Durham Probate Records. Inventory of John Heath, 1639/40.
89. *Memorials,* 136 and note 1; PSA *(Newcastle),* 3rd series, III (1889), 432 (both cup and cover paten are hall-marked for 1638); Surtees IV (11), 39; *VCH Durham,* III, 189.
90. *Wills,* II, 207-9; DRO D/Lo/F 270; DRO D/Lo/F 321; DRO D/X 790/1, 87-9. It is likely that the Heaths lived in the parish of St Mary-le-Bow, as Elizabeth Heath was baptised in the church there, 12 October 1626, see DRO EP/Du MB 1, and John Heath was the churchwarden in 1637 (Hutchinson, II, 289 note).

91. DRO D/Lo/F 270; E. Mackenzie and M. Ross, *View of the County Palatine of Durham* (1834), 394; *Memorials,* 136; Surtees IV (11), 58, 59, 66 and note p, 91, 92; *VCH Durham*, III, 166-7.
92. *PSA (Newcastle)*, (as note 86 above), 433; Surtees IV (11), 92; *VCH Durham*, 167, 189.
93. *VCH Durham*, II, 168-71, 236; R. Welford, op.cit., xvii, xviii, 162-3 and notes, 168.
94. R. Welford, *op.cit.,* 20-1.
95. G. Ornsby (ed.), *The Correspondence of John Cosin*, vol. II (SS 55, 1872), 217.
96. *Memorials,* 128 and note 1, 129, 143; Surtees IV (11), 66-7; *VCH Durham*, III, 185.
97. Surtees IV (11), 67; *VCH Durham*, III, 185.
98. C. Morris (ed.), *The Journeys of Celia Fiennes* (The Cresset Press, London, 1947), 215-6.
99. Durham Probate Records. Will of William Robinson of Kepier, gardener, 1757; *The Durham Chronicle,* 3 August 1883, 'Local Sketches'.
100. R.M. Clay, *op.cit.,* 91-3; Everett and Masterman, *op.cit.,* 26 and Table C; James Rush, *A Beilby Odyssey* (Nelson and Saunders, Olney, Buckinghamshire, 1987), 47, 50, 120 no. 85 (wrongly titled 'Brinkburn Abbey on the Coquet'). I am grateful to Mr Martin Roberts for bringing this water-colour to my attention. The entrance into the close was blocked in the 1950s (Mrs Ruth Watson).
101. *History, Directory, and Gazetteer, of the Counties of Durham and Northumberland.* . . . (Parson and White, Newcastle, 1827), I, 204; Everett and Masterman, *op.cit.,* 11, 32. Two descendants of Mary Pearson, sister of the brothers, Alastair Rose and his sister, Ann Greenwood, of New Zealand, visited Kepier and St Giles' church in June 1993.
102. Information from Mrs Linda Drury.
103. D D (1871), 46.
104. Durham Probate Records, Will of John Banks of Kepier Mill, 1702; Mackenzie and Ross, *op.cit.,* II, 394.
105. *Memorials,* 159. John Coulson had been a witness to the will of John Banks; D D (1871), 46.
106. *The Durham Chronicle*, 30 September 1870.
107. *The Durham Chronicle*, 3 August 1883, 'Local Sketches'; Surtees IV (11), 92; DRO D/Lo/P 75.
108. *D D, passim; DCYB,* passim: David J. Butler, *Durham City: The 1851 Census* (Durham Historical Enterprises, Durham, 1992), 170.
109. *PSA (Newcastle)*, NS III (1889), 139-40.
110. Note by F.W. Morgan in his Sketch Book 15 (at RIBA). Thanks are due to Professor G.R. Batho and Mr M.F. Richardson for bringing the Morgan sketch-books to my notice.

111. June Crosby, *Durham in Old Photographs* (Alan Sutton, Stroud, 1990), 74.
112. Taylor-Wilson, page headed, 'Kepier House: the structural condition of the ruin'.
113. *VCH Durham*, I, 393; II, 115. The caption about 'Jack' was seen at the centenary exhibition of Durham Photographic Society (section by Durham City Arts) at the Durham Light Infantry Museum, October 1992.
114. *D D*, passim; *DCYB*, passim. Information about tenancy and ownership from Mrs Ruth Watson, the present owner of Kepier. Information about the proposed power station from Mrs June Crosby, Deputy-chairman of the City of Durham Trust.